Daniel Lewis

Cancer, and its treatment

Daniel Lewis

Cancer, and its treatment

ISBN/EAN: 9783337714819

Printed in Europe, USA, Canada, Australia, Japan

Cover: Foto ©ninafisch / pixelio.de

More available books at **www.hansebooks.com**

CANCER,

AND ITS TREATMENT.

BY

DANIEL LEWIS, A.M., M.D., Ph.D.,

Surgeon to the New York Skin and Cancer Hospital; Professor of Surgery (Cancerous Diseases) in the New York Post-Graduate Medical School.

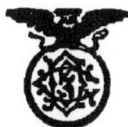

GEORGE S. DAVIS,
DETROIT, MICH.

CONTENTS.

ı

ı

PREFACE.

This volume contains the essential features of the course of clinical lectures delivered at the New York Post-Graduate Medical School on the subject of Cancer. The deductions here published are based upon the study of 534 cases, occurring in my service at the New York Skin and Cancer Hospital and in private practice. Within such narrow limits it is impossible to include even a synopsis of the entire subject of Cancer, and, therefore, the discussion has been limited chiefly to such topics as bear directly upon the successful treatment of certain forms of the disease.

Some comparatively new methods of treatment are described, as well as modifications of usual methods in the management of certain cases, which have been proved to be valuable. The employment of caustic applications has received considerable attention, and the cases in which their use is advisable, as well as those in which such means of treatment are inadmissible, have been indicated.

It has been my purpose to reiterate the importance of making an early diagnosis, to be followed by prompt and radical efforts to remove the disease, even in the pre-cancerous stage, with the firm conviction that the appreciation of this necessity by both patients and physicians will soon place Cancer in the list of curable diseases.

D. L.

249 Madison Ave., New York,
    February, 1892.

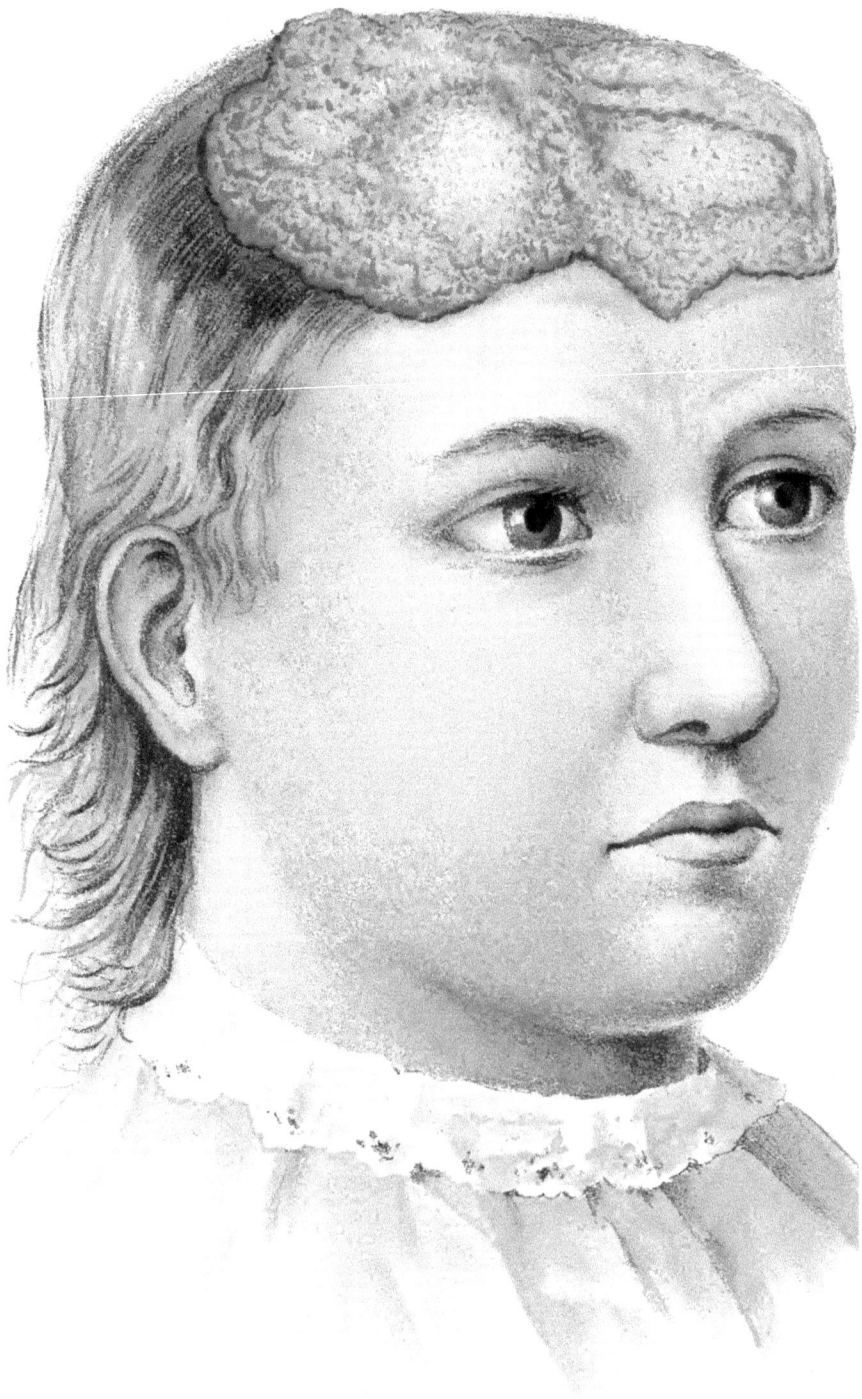

SARCOMA OF THE SCALP.

CANCER AND ITS TREATMENT.

CHAPTER I.

DEFINITION—MEDICINAL AGENTS—CHIAN TUR-PENTINE—CHLORIDE OF ANILINE—PYOK-TANIN—DR. SNOW'S CLASSIFICATION.

The term cancer is a convenient one for general use, provided we have a uniform understanding as to its application. In the following pages all malignant neoplasms are denominated cancer.

Dr. Herbert L. Snow has given the following characteristics of cancer:*

1. Resistance to all known medicinal agents.

2. Proneness to invade other organs and tissues of the body than those in which it has originated.

3. Liability to recur after removal by caustics or the surgeon's knife.

4. The pain to which it commonly gives rise.

5. The tendency to destroy life.

Although there are widely varying degrees of malignancy, depending upon the condition of the patient, the location of the disease, and the variety of the structure of the tumor itself, yet all will agree that

---

* Clinical Notes on Cancer.

the characters enumerated, when found in a given case, are sufficient for the clinical diagnosis of cancer. The researches of the microscopist have determined with some degree of accuracy the minute anatomy of the different varieties of malignant growths, but the fact remains that the surgeon must almost invariably base his treatment upon the gross appearances and clinical history.

The first characteristic named, "resistance to all known medicinal agents," may in the near future be modified by the experiments now being made with new medicinal agents. A brief review of our experience with some of them may be profitably considered.

I. CHIAN TURPENTINE.

This remedy, the internal administration of which as a remedy for cancer has recently been recommended anew by Professor John Clay, obstetric surgeon to the Queen's Hospital, Birmingham, England, is a product of the *Pistacia terebinthus*, a tree which in its native island of Scio, in the Mediterranean, grows to the height of thirty or forty feet. The gum is obtained from incisions into the bark, and the many impurities which it contains are composed of sand, leaves, straw, and particles of the bark and fruit. As Professor Clay insists that its efficiency depends upon the genuineness of the drug, it is well to carefully consider the following description from Flückiger and Hanbury's "Pharmacographia":

"Chian turpentine, as found in commerce and believed to be genuine, is a soft solid, becoming brittle by exposure to the air; viewed in mass, it appears opaque and of a dull brown hue. If pressed while warm between two slips of glass, it is seen to be transparent, of a yellowish brown, and much contaminated by various impurities in a state of fine division. It has an agreeable, mild terebinthinous odor, *and very little taste.* The whitish powder with which old Chian turpentine becomes covered shows no trace of crystalline structure when examined under the microscope."

It is believed that Strassburg and Venice turpentine and Canada balsam are often substituted for it, which can easily be detected by applying the tests as to taste, odor, and appearance given above.

The turpentine, as used by Clay in his first reported cases,* was given in the form of a pill, containing three grains, combined with two grains of flowers of sulphur. Two of these pills were given every four hours for many weeks, and in some cases for nearly a year. It was found that in some instances the turpentine in the pill form was not well digested, and the latest recommendation of Professor Clay is to administer it in the form of an emulsion made as follows:

One ounce of the Chian turpentine is to be dissolved in two ounces of sulphuric ether. This solu-

---

* Lancet, March 27th, 1880.

tion has been termed the turpentine essence, and the emulsion is made by adding one ounce of this essence to a mucilage of acacia (one ounce and a half of powdered gum Arabic and water to nine ounces), making a ten-ounce mixture, a teaspoonful of which contains about three grains of the drug. A dessert-spoonful, it will be observed, contains the same amount of turpentine as the two pills which were previously recommended. In some cases resorcin has been added in doses of a grain. This emulsion is not of a disagreeable taste, as nearly all of my patients who are under the treatment testify.

Tonics have been used when indicated. In some instances local applications have been made, in others this internal remedy alone has been employed. When it has been taken for about three months it should be omitted three days in every fortnight. The sulphur is often given in a separate pill, especially in cancer of the uterus and rectum. I have given this description of the plan in order that we may have an accurate knowledge of what this Chian turpentine treatment really is.

We are all familiar with the statements which Professor Clay has repeatedly made concerning its efficacy. He has seen a number of complete cures, not only of uterine cancer in advanced stages, but also of cancer of the rectum and surface epitheliomata. In cancer of the breast he reports marked improvement of symptoms and complete arrest of the new growth.

No report has yet been published, as far as I can learn, stating the precise changes in the tumor, but he maintains that the primary action is upon the periphery of the growth. The plan has been tested in the London Cancer Hospital, and, after a tolerably thorough trial, condemned by Dr. Marsden and Mr. Purcell. Another trial has recently been made, however, and one of the surgeons of the same hospital declares the Chian turpentine to be a very useful remedy in many cases.

Several patients in my service in the New York Skin and Cancer Hospital were placed upon the treatment early in 1888, and it was faithfully followed in eight of them for periods varying from three months to two years. Two were uterine cases; one of these was not affected in the slightest degree.

The other came into the hospital with extensive ulceration of the cervix. There were three nodules in the vaginal wall, evidently cancerous. The patient was anæmic, sleepless, irritable; hæmorrhage was of daily occurrence, and pain almost constant. Without the employment of any local treatment except carbolized douches, in twelve weeks the hæmorrhage and pain had ceased entirely, the vaginal nodules had become soft, and the ulcer of the cervix was half its original size and seemed to be a healthy granulating surface. The patient believed she was well, and we were unable to prevent her return to her home. Three months afterward she was re-admitted with the disease again active, and nothing impeded its fatal progress. It seemed certain that the marked improvement in the first instance was due to the drug, and I regret exceedingly that the experiment was interrupted.

One patient with extensive epithelioma of the face showed decided arrest of the ulceration, and general improvement in symptoms, as well as in the appearance of the diseased surface. No absolute cures were effected, but I yet employ it in some cases, believing that it is of sufficient value to hold a place in our meagre list of internal remedies for cancer.

2. CHLORIDE OF ANILINE.

In June, 1891, my attention was called to the chloride of aniline by Dr. C. E. Bruce of New York, who had observed a marked improvement in a cancer of the tongue following hypodermic injections of from ten to twenty drops of a ten-per-cent. solution (in dilute alcohol) repeated about twice a week. The injection had been made in the arm or between the shoulders, and when carefully done produced no disagreeable effects. After a few weeks' treatment, pain was relieved, infiltration was diminished to such an extent that the patient could protrude the tongue (which was an impossibility before the injections were commenced), and swallowing became much easier.

A laboring man, aged 55, entered my service at the Skin and Cancer Hospital six months ago with an epithelioma of the tongue on the right side, about one and a-half inches from the tip. At the border it was ulcerated, and the hardened tissue beneath the tongue was continuous with a new growth the size of a robin's egg, which protruded below the body of the inferior maxilla. Pain was a prominent symptom, and swallowing was both painful and difficult. Had this case followed the usual course, its destructive influence would have destroyed the patient's life within a year. Under the steady use of the chloride of aniline injections the ulcer has not increased in size, the tumor under the jaw is smaller, he takes food as well as upon admission, and the entire course of the disease has been favorably modified.

Some decrease in induration, and improvement in mobility of the arm, has been noted in an inoperable recurrent tumor of the right breast, in a case which we have had under treatment for six weeks, and there seems sufficient ground for persevering in its employment.

Some German observers have reported favorable results with this drug, and some have condemned it. No authentic records of absolute cure have been published. It seems fair to say, however, that there is some ground for the hypothesis that the drug acts upon the cell elements of these neoplasms through the blood corpuscles. It has no detrimental influence upon the general health of the patient, and causes no febrile reaction. In other words, its use is devoid of all danger. We should continue our experiments, not without hope of satisfactory results in some cases.

3. PYOKTANIN.

Professor von Mosetig, of Vienna, published a paper in January, 1891,* reporting his experience with pyoktanin, in which he claimed some good results from injections of a solution of 1 to 1000. Since that time many reports from other observers, both at home and abroad, have appeared in medical journals, and it is evident that in many instances the growth of the tumors has been checked. Some fatal accidents have occurred which have been attributed to the drug, so that pyoktanin, methylene blue, fuchsin, and the other aniline dyes, should be cautiously employed. In the New York Hospital experiments with these drugs have been abandoned, as well as in the Skin and Cancer Hospital. As with the chloride solutions, however, so with the others; enough has been secured to suggest bright possibilities, and therefore mention has been made of these remedies. *In no instance, however, should such means be employed where a complete removal of the diseased tissue can be secured by operative procedure.*

In closing this introductory chapter, a classification of cancer from Dr. Snow's work, already referred to, is appended, as furnishing the most satisfactory arrangement of such diseases thus far published for clinical study. As an aid to correct *prognosis*, all tumors should be classified by microscopical exami-

---

* Wiener Klinische Wochenschrift, 1891, No. 6.

nation after removal, but in regard to *treatment* no delusive pathological report should ever hinder us from removing by some means any new growth which exhibits even a tendency to malignancy.

MR. SNOW'S CLASSIFICATION OF CANCER.

I.

ALVEOLAR CARCINOMA. $\quad$ (*a*) Scirrhus.

(Derived from glandular epithelium, characterized by locular structure).

(*b*) Encephaloid. $\begin{cases} \text{(Sub-variety).} \\ \text{Colloid.} \end{cases}$

II.

SARCOMA.

(Origin from connective tissue corpuscles. No locular structure).

Round-celled.
Spindle-celled $\begin{cases} \text{Sub-} \\ \text{varieties} \end{cases}$ $\begin{cases} \text{Osteoid.} \\ \text{Melanoid.} \end{cases}$
Mixed.
Glioma.
Myaloid.

III.

EPITHELIOMA. $\quad$ (*a*) Scaly.

(Proliferation of epithelium on skin or mucous membrane).

(*b*) Columnar. $\begin{cases} \text{(Sub-variety).} \\ \text{Duct Cancer.} \end{cases}$

IV.

LYMPHADENOMA.

(Proliferation of lymphatic gland elements).

CHAPTER II.

DEVELOPMENT OF CANCER FROM NON-MALIG-NANT DISEASES—WARTS—MOLES—SEBA-CEOUS TUMORS—SIMPLE ULCERS—SYPHILITIC ULCERS—PHIMO-SIS—UMBILICAL HERNIA.

Any course of treatment for the cure of cancer is successful in proportion to the extent of the disease and its location; but to a greater extent to its duration from the first appearance of the diseased condition. Mr. Jonathan Hutchinson read a paper on the "Origin of Tumors," before the British Medical Association,[*] in which he describes what he aptly designates the "pre-cancerous stage," which probably is present in every instance, although often overlooked when it happens to be of short duration. If the purely local origin of cancer be accepted as the correct theory, and Sir James Paget is now the only conspicuous advocate of the old "constitutional origin" notion, there is a period in the history of every case when the treatment of a disease not truly cancerous would insure curative results not hitherto attained. With this idea in view a number of cases are here noted of non-malignant diseases which have been observed to be precursors of cancer.

---

[*] Transactions of the British Medical Association, 1882.

1. WARTS.

In a paper published in the American Practitioner for December, 1874,* I gave a brief report of a case (No. 1) occurring in a man fifty-five years of age, who had a small wart on the right side of the nose, about three-quarters of an inch from the angle of the eye, which had existed many years, without showing any sign of malignancy. Two years before its removal it became slightly ulcerated, without any known cause, and from that time forward it increased gradually in size until at the end of the two years it was an unmistakable epithelioma. The cervical glands were considerably enlarged. It was removed by Marsden's arsenical mucilage, and healed completely; but the patient died two years later of cancer of the left lung.

Dr. Thin relates a case of rodent ulcer (epithelioma), which began four years before its final removal by operation, as a little wart by the side of the nose, the lip of that side being at the same time swollen, on account of inflammation of the eye-tooth.

It increased in size very slowly, and three years after its commencement caustic was applied, which seemed to improve it at first; but it soon began to increase rapidly, and when removed, twelve months later, it was an ulcer one-half inch by an inch.

---

*Read before the Medical Society of the County of New York, June, 1874.

Microscopical examination of sections through the border and surface of the ulcer exhibited the usual cell arrangement of rodent ulcer.

In both of these cases there is no history of heredity, and in my own case the history is authentic for at least two generations.

2. MOLES.

Numerous instances are recorded in which the ordinary mole became the seat of cancerous disease.

Mr. H. Thompson reported the following case at a meeting of the London Pathological Society, November 6th, 1860:

A lady, aged sixty, was subject from birth to a small black mole on the outer side of the left arm.

It became irritated in hot weather for two summers, the second time remaining red and swollen, and a melanoid cancer of the size of a large nut resulted, which was attended with a large glandular tumor in the axilla of the same side.

It seems that the melanoid variety of cancer chooses the neighborhood of a congenital mole, or wart, for its development, as in the instance just related.

Mr. Pemberton, of the Birmingham General Hospital, in his work on cancer, emphasizes this point, and one of his cases is so characteristic that I will give it as he relates it:

"Mrs. M. H., aged forty-five, had several congenital moles on different parts of the body, one of which was near the middle of the forearm.

"Ulceration began around its edge first, and spread therefrom, leaving the mole untouched. At the end of four years, an irregular ulcer, two inches in its longest diameter, was produced, with borders elevated, dark-colored, and indurated.

" The entire portion was removed by operation down to the muscles beneath, and, four years later, she remained well. There were no enlarged glands, and no history of cancer in the family."

Other varieties of cancer than the melanoid often develop in moles, however, and the same author (Pemberton) relates several cases where an irritation or slight injury of a congenital mole was followed by the encephaloid variety.

3.—SEBACEOUS TUMORS.

Sebaceous tumors often result in cancer after they have existed for long periods without showing any malignant tendency. Sometimes, when middle life is reached and the tendency to degenerative changes is at its maximum, these growths will begin to show signs of activity; some tenderness and pain, less mobility, and a thickening of the walls near the base of the tumor are often among the first changes noted. Ulceration follows later, and the course of the disease thenceforth does not differ from that of cancer from other causes.

Injuries play an important part in other cases; and the following case, occurring in the practice of Dr. W. W. Crandall, of Wellsville, N. Y., will furnish an excellent illustration:

A man, aged fifty-five, with a wen on the vertex, one inch and a half in its longest diameter, which had existed for a score of years or more, accidentally struck it against a sharp piece of wood, which, if I remember rightly, caused slight bleeding. Inflammation of the tumor followed, then ulceration and sloughing, which was followed, after a few weeks, by cancerous disease of the entire border and base of the ulcer. It was finally removed by Marsden's method, and the history was published in the paper above mentioned. There was no family history of cancer.

Mr. C. Aston Key has reported a case of sebaceous tumor of the scalp * which he removed from the scalp of a lady sixty-nine years of age. The top of the tumor had sloughed, the margin of the opening assumed a cancerous character, and, after the whole tumor was removed, a quantity of glairy fluid was found at its lower portion, having all the physical appearance of colloid. Family history not mentioned.

4.—SIMPLE ULCERS.

Simple ulcers occasionally become malignant, and two very interesting cases of that kind were

---

*Trans. London Path. Soc. Vol. i, p. 345.

under treatment at the New York Skin and Cancer Hospital, in the service of Dr. Bulkley, in 1882.

The first was that of a woman, aged fifty-five, who fell down a flight of stairs six years before, receiving several cuts about the face by corners of zinc covering the steps. All healed except one on the right ala nasi, which continued to discharge a little watery fluid, and occasionally form a scab over it, until within a year and a half, when it began to increase in size quite rapidly and became nearly two square inches in extent, and an unmistakable epithelioma. A second subsequently developed just below the left eye, and entirely distinct from the first ulcer. The patient was positive in her statement that no cancer had ever occurred in her family.

The second case was in a man, fifty-seven years of age, who received an abrasion of the skin on the left leg thirty years before, which healed in a few weeks. Ever since that time, however, he had often complained of severe itching on the site of the injury, and scratching it abraded the skin, and quite a large ulcer had often been the result. It had not been healed for about six years; and during an acute attack of rheumatism, two years before, it began to increase in size, and, notwithstanding all the remedies applicable to such cases had been employed for its cure, it steadily advanced. The history, upon admission to the hospital, was as follows:

"It is now a deep, irregular ulcer, extending

from the ankle nine inches up the leg, its lateral
diameter being about seven inches.

"The surface is covered with irregular nodules
and furrows, of a dark red color, and secreting a considerable watery fluid. The edges are elevated and
indurated for nearly an inch from the border, and,
when compressed firmly, exude a little fluid resembling pus. The entire ulcer is the seat of an almost
constant burning pain, described by the patient like
the sensation of having boiling water poured over it.

"The man has been a coachman for thirty years,
and was never sick. Even now his general appearance indicates good health. There is a bare possibility of heredity, as one brother died from some
'sore' a few years ago."

An authentic case of cancer developed from an
innocent ulcer is reported by Mr. Jonathan Hutchinson:*

"The patient was a woman, aged sixty, who had
suffered from onychia of the right great toe for about
eight months. It was said to have been caused by a
tight shoe. When the remnants of dead nail were
removed, the matrix and adjacent parts were in an
inflamed and very irritable state, and resisted all
efforts to heal them. The base of the ulcer became
gradually thicker and more swollen, and syphilis
being suspected, iodide of potassium was adminis-
tered, but without benefit.

---

* Transactions of the London Path. Soc. Vol. viii, p. 404.

" Induration increased and pain became more severe, and of a darting, pricking character.

" Enlarged glands were then discovered about the middle of the thigh, just over the large vessels where Mr. Hutchinson has several times observed the first glandular enlargement in melanosis of the foot. The glands of the groin were not affected. The toe was removed, and found to be the seat of melanotic and medullary cancer."

At that time the woman had not materially lost flesh, and was in good health, although the trouble had existed two years. Eight months later she returned with a bleeding mass of cancer in the groin, and also recurrent disease in the stump of the toe. In this case also there was no history of hereditary cancer.

5. SYPHILITIC ULCERS.

Syphilis is often the direct cause of cancer, especially when the disease appears as a chronic ulcer of the tongue. The extreme difficulty of curing these syphilitic sores by the ordinary treatment is doubtless familiar to every practitioner.

I have recently seen a syphilitic patient, who had been under treatment in hospital for several months with ulceration of the tongue, develop an affection of the parotid and sublingual glands of the same side, which was undoubtedly malignant.

Walsh does not admit that syphilis is a cause of

2 DDD

cancer,* and brings forward arguments against it, the chief one being that it is a rare disease among prostitutes, in whom syphilis is presumably quite common. This argument loses its force when the age of that class is considered, the average of which is much below that at which cancer most frequently occurs.

Scirrhus of the penis has been observed to spring from a syphilitic sore, and even Walsh says: "Venereal ulcers may become complicated by carcinomatous deposition and fungate in the same manner as primary cancer." The same authority also declares that venereal warts may terminate in cancer.

6. PHIMOSIS.

Cancer of the penis has been so frequently observed associated with congenital phimosis that many writers have placed it among the causes of the disease, and the retention of the natural secretions is believed to be the exciting cause. Ten patients out of twelve, treated for cancer of the penis by Hey, had either congenital or acquired phimosis.

7. UMBILICAL HERNIA.

Under this head is given the history of what I believe to be a unique case, but one which illustrates in a marked degree the result of prolonged local

---

* "The Nature and Treatment of Cancer," pp. 155 and 408.

irritation as a cause of cancer. The case has been reported by me to the Medical Society of the county of New York.*

Mrs. B——, a widow, aged sixty-seven years, had suffered from umbilical hernia fifteen years, but had never worn a truss, having always reduced the protruding intestine easily and frequently, until about a year before applying to me for treatment.

She then began to suffer pain about the umbilicus, and so much soreness that for the three preceding months she had not attempted to replace the tumor. The pain increased rapidly, and radiated to the stomach and pelvic regions, and a marked failure in flesh and strength, frequent vomiting, constipation alternating with diarrhœa, sleeplessness, and fever compelled her to seek advice.

A monthly metrorrhagia of more or less severity had excited no especial surprise in the patient's mind, although continued more than twenty-five years beyond the usual period.

Upon examining the supposed hernia, I found a hard, nodulated tumor of a bluish-red color, the surface of which was slightly ulcerated, in the fold of skin at the upper portion. It extended nearly an inch beyond the border of the hernial ring, seemed quite movable with the skin, and it was a hope shared by Dr. A. N. Brockway, who saw the case with me,

---

* N. Y. Medical Record, Oct. 12, 1889.

that the disease had not invaded the peritoneal cavity. An operation was advised, and after the patient was etherized, so that a thorough examination of the base of the tumor could be made, it was found to invade the ring, and all hope of a slight operation was abandoned. An elliptical incision being made, the tumor was dissected out as far as the ring, and then carefully examined for any intestinal contents. It evidently contained no gut, and was removed in order to facilitate examination of the parts beneath. The sac contained some omentum which was not diseased. The subperitoneal tissue was infiltrated as far as the finger could reach. It was thoroughly removed, and the wound then closed as after ovariotomy.

The patient rallied well after the operation, but died sixty hours afterward, apparently from shock, no peritonitis having developed.

It should be stated that an examination, while the patient was under ether, revealed a much enlarged cervix, but no sign of cancer, although the body of the uterus was so large as to suggest the possibility of its being the seat of malignant disease.

The first section from the apex of the tumor proved to be a large, round-celled, alveolar sarcoma.

The second section was from a portion of the base of the tumor just outside the neck of the sac, and was of especial interest on account of the gland-tissue which it contained, the origin of which was believed to be embryonic.

Dr. George T. Elliot has very kindly furnished me the following description of this rare form of tumor:

"The portions of the tumor removed from the umbilical region, which were received by me for microscopical examination, were hardened in alcohol, and the sections were stained with borax-carmin and pyrogallic acid and iron.

"It was not difficult to determine the nature of the growth, since portions of the sections were found composed of small spindle-shaped cells, with here and there a few large round cells, while in others these latter were arranged in more or less large alveoli formed by the bundles of connective tissue. In many of these alveoli, capillary blood-vessels, which were abundant throughout the tissue, penetrated in between the cells contained in them. From these features it was evident that the new-growth was a sarcoma composed of mixed cells, spindle-shaped and round.

"In addition to the sarcomatous tissue, however, there were found other histological elements which greatly increased the interest taken in the specimen. Distributed throughout the sections, more or less abundantly, glandular tissue was found, which was in every way identical with the glands of Lieberkuhn existing in the small intestines.

" The glands were composed of a basement membrane and columnar epithelium, and they were separated one from another by more or less connective or sarcomatous tissue. Some were unchanged, others were hyperplastic, while still others had·undergone cystic degeneration.

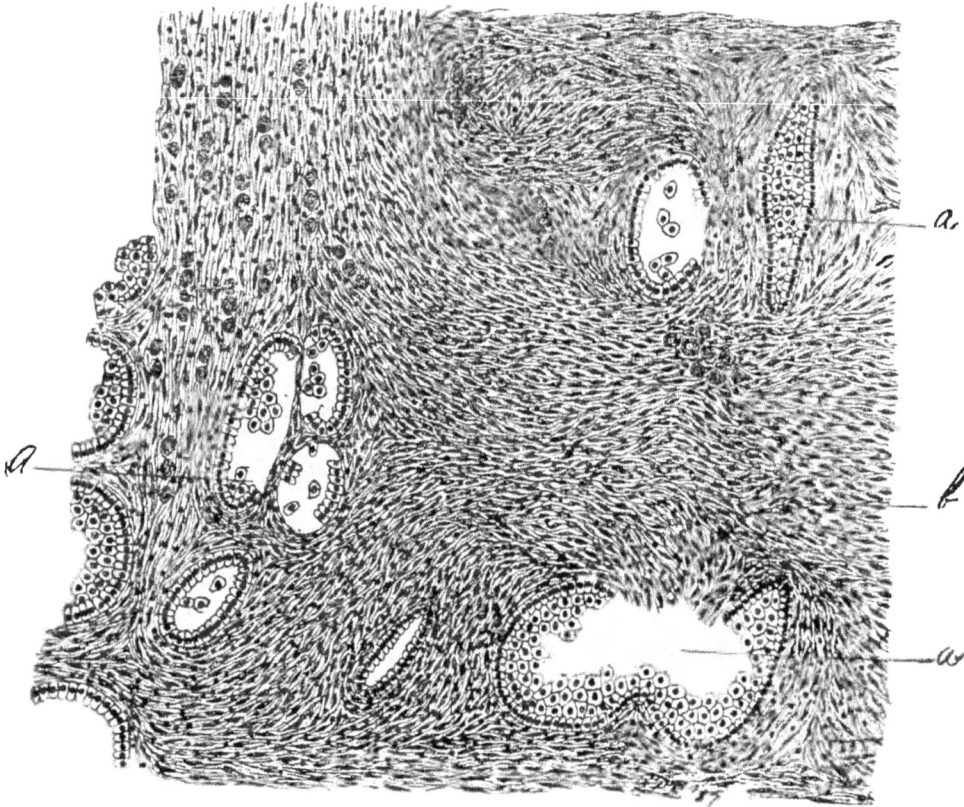

A—Glandular tissue more or less surrounded by small spindle-celled (b) sarcomatous tissue, and large round sarcoma-cell.

" The tissue between them was more or less infiltrated with small round infiltration-cells.

" The presence of the intestinal glandular tissue in this tumor is not an extraordinary fact, but yet one

which is rarely met with.   Growths of this class occur
at the umbilicus, and are known under the name of
enteroteratoma.   To understand the occurrence of
these growths, it must be remembered that in fœtal
life the ductus omphalo-mesentericus is prolonged
into the umbilical cord, but normally disappears
before birth.   Abnormally, however, it may persist

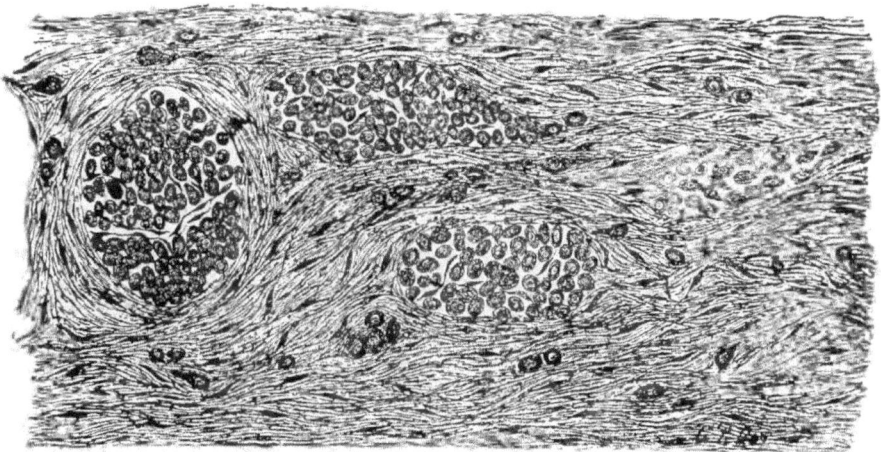

Alveolar large round cell sarcoma.   Section through tumor
at its apex.

and develop into a tube resembling intestine, and
either form a congenital diverticulum of the small
intestines, or more rarely, if this development has
occurred in the portion of the duct situated just in
front of the navel, there remains a small tumor after
the falling off of the severed umbilical cord.

"This seems to be the only way in which the
presence of the intestinal glands in the tumor could

be explained; that is, that the original growth was an enteroteratoma to which no attention had been paid, but which persisted and finally underwent sarcomatous degeneration. It seems, however, remarkable that it should have persisted so long before undergoing change."

CHAPTER III.

DEVELOPMENT OF CANCER FROM NON-MALIG NANT DISEASES—PSORIASIS—ICHTHYOSIS OF THE TONGUE—LEUCOPLAKIA— ECZEMA, OR PAGET'S DISEASE OF THE NIPPLE—REMARKS ON THE ÆTIOLOGY OF CANCER.

8. PSORIASIS.

At least four cases are now on record where epithelioma has developed on a psoriatic base—two by Dr. White in 1885, one by Cartay in 1878, and one by Hebra.

In White's and Hebra's cases there was a transition of warty growth of the plaques, a form to which the name of psoriasis verrucosa is given. These cases, while showing that psoriasis is not simply a parakeratosis, but also of inflammatory nature, renders a prognosis of much greater moment in cases where any appearance of warty growth is manifested.

Under this head may be mentioned the so-called ichthyosis of the tongue, which in a certain proportion of cases has been observed to terminate in epithelioma or carcinoma. Without undertaking any criticism or justification of this application of the term ichthyosis, I will simply say that reference is made to such cases as Mr. Hulke, of the Middlesex Hospital, described before the Clinical Society of London a few years ago under that name. In one case, which terminated in fatal carcinoma, there was an area of disease over which the papillæ were greatly hypertrophied; the surface of that part of the dorsum was warty on account of the overgrowth of the papillæ, which, instead of preserving their natural consistence, were much harder than natural and sometimes quite "horny." There were three such patches, which were removed by operation, but the cancerous disease developed from smaller patches which were not removed, and not in the cicatrices, which remained healthy.

Leucoma, or leucoplakia, sometimes terminates in malignant disease. I have recently removed by operation an epithelioma of the lower lip in a man of forty (who was not a smoker), which began as a leucoplakia of the inside and border of the lip.

9. ECZEMA, OR PAGET'S DISEASE OF THE NIPPLE.

The development of cancer of the breast, when a chronic eczema of the nipple had existed for a long time, has naturally led to the inference that they stood in the relation of cause and effect.

Mr Henry Morris, of the Middlesex Hospital, reported two cases, in one of which the eruption existed four years, and in the other six, before cancer was suspected. Both patients died of secondary cancer.

Mr. Thomas W. Nunn, in his recent admirable

work on " Cancer of the Breast," refers to Mr. Morris' cases in connection with one observed by himself, and also furnishes the conclusions arrived at by Mr. H. T. Butlin, in a paper on the same subject.

I take the liberty of copying Mr. Butlin's propositions as Mr. Nunn gives them:

1. That a certain relation existed between the eczema of the nipple and the areola and the carcinoma of the breast.

2. That one of the first effects of the eczema was to produce proliferation of the mucous layer of the epidermis of the parts affected.

3. That in time the epithelium lining the galactophorous ducts became affected in like manner.

4. That the disease, traveling along the large ducts, reached the smaller ducts and acini, which became dilated and filled with proliferating epithelium, which was at length, so to speak, discharged into the surrounding tissues.

5. That the carcinoma thus formed was therefore essentially a disease of epithelium.

Whether we accept this theory of production, or the opposing one of Dr. Thin—that, instead of a cell proliferation, the growth is the result of a special development of colorless blood corpuscles—the fact that cancer of the breast does result from eczema of the nipple and areola seems to be pretty well established.

---

*Med. Chirurg. Trans., Vol. LXIII, p. 37.

This disease is known in literature as Paget's Disease of the Nipple, because it was first described by Sir James Paget.* (See illustration opposite p. 32.)

His report was based upon fourteen cases, in patients varying from 40 to 60 years of age. The nipple, or areola, or both, in some instances, were observed to be the seat of an intensely red, very granular, raw surface, discharging a copious, clear, yellowish, viscid fluid, and attended with a tingling, itching or burning sensation.

In some of the cases the eruption was dry like psoriasis, while in others only the ordinary characters of chronic eczema were presented.

Dr. S. W. Gross accepts the view of Sir James Paget that these cases are simple eczema in the beginning, and from the long-continued irritation produce cancer, just as the ichthyosis of the tongue has been shown to produce epithelioma of that organ.

This view is supported by the authentic reports of cure of such an eruption of the nipple by Busch, and also by Dr. Gross, who successfully treated such a chronic eczema by a lotion composed of equal parts of glycerin and laudanum.

I have had two cases in which cancer developed, the diagnosis of which was verified by the microscope after amputation of the breast. The eczema involved only one nipple.

---

* Report of St. Bartholomew Hospital, Vol. X, p. 87.

Another case was cured by resorcin ointment and a general tonic treatment, although the disease had persisted for eighteen months, which proves that Mr. Lawson's advice to excise any breast where eczema of the nipple resists treatment for one year is not to be implicitly followed in all cases. No recurrence has occurred in my cases after three years, and it seems to be true that this paricular variety of cancer of the breast is less malignant than the usual form of the disease.

Numerous cases similar to those here presented are recorded, but enough have been cited, I believe, to establish beyond question that cancer is not always the outgrowth of malignancy. In other words, in the cases here recorded there was a pre-cancerous stage, when the patient could have been cured by removing a simple subaceous tumor or a wart—by a judicious management of an eczema of the nipple, or a lacerated wound of the face.

Any long continued irritation, such as a broken tooth upon the lip or tongue, inflamed hæmorrhoids, or chronic inflammation in a lacerated cervix uteri, will very often cause cancer.

In such local causes are to be found the most important factors in the ætiology of malignant diseases. Heredity plays so insignificant a part in causation that it may be left out of future consideration. Less than five per cent. of my five hundred cases gave any family history of cancer whatever. In most instances where two or more cases have occurred in a family it is simply a coincidence, just as it is where two or more near relatives die of pneumonia.

Until the pathologist discovers a cancer bacillus, we must continue to affirm that the causes we have referred to in this and the preceding chapter are sufficient to produce the disease in such organs as the age and general condition of the patient may have rendered susceptible to such epithelial degenerations.

Before leaving this subject permit me to enter a strong protest against the common practice of trying the effect of mild caustics, such as nitrate of silver, pyrogallic acid, resorcin, and many others, upon these malignant diseases. Nearly always such applications stimulate the progress of the disease, and very seldom do any good whatever. This is eminently true of the galvanic current as applied to the surface of tumors.

A scirrhous tumor of the breast, which the physician in charge permitted me to examine recently, had made such remarkably rapid progress that some special cause was sought for, and found, as I believe, in the mild and frequently repeated galvanization of the tumor by an over-zealous advocate of that remedy.

CHAPTER IV.

REMARKS ON DIAGNOSIS—CLINICAL FEATURES
SUFFICIENT—MICROSCOPICAL EXAMINA-
TION VALUABLE FOR PROGNOSIS—
IN DOUBTFUL CASES TREAT
THE DISEASE AS
CANCER.

Success or failure in the treatment of cancer depends largely upon an *early* diagnosis. Every surgeon who sees many patients is familiar with the dis-
heartening recital of the patient that she showed the
tumor to her family physician months ago, who advised the use of some ointment or other local application, and told her to inform him if it did not disap-
pear. I cannot hold the physician blameless who
thus calms a patient's anxiety by what he knows, or
should know, to be utterly false advice, for which his
unfortunate patient often pays with her life

The references already made to the diseases
which are often the exciting cause of cancer should
emphasize the necessity for a most careful and consci-
entious study of any and every new growth in every
case, and especially in those where the patient has
reached forty years of age. I have now under treatment the most malignant disease of the orbit I have
ever seen, and the boy is only nine years old; but
fortunately cancer in early life is a rare affection. It

is pre-eminently a disease of middle life. This is especially true of cancer of the female breast, which, from its frequency, may be taken as the type of the disease for purposes of study.

Dr. Willard Parker's table of 359 cases of cancer of the breast* is exceedingly valuable as showing the age at which the development is most frequent. Of his cases the disease commenced—

Between 25 and 30 years, in...................... 5 cases
"   30   " 35   "   "   23   "
"   35   " 40   "   "   54   "
"   40   " 45   "   "   78   "
"   45   " .50   "   "   80   "
"   50   " 55   "   "   57   "
"   55   " 60   "   "   31   "
"   60   " 65   "   "   12   "
"   65   " 70   "   "   14   "
"   70   " 80   "   "   5   "

                                                      ———
                                                      359

It thus appears that 246, or more than 68 per cent. of the entire number, began between the ages of 40 and 60, while only 82, or 22 per cent., were between 25 and 40, and of these 5 cases only were under 30 years of age. My own tables and all others show about the same proportions, so that we may place the age of the patient among the most important elements of diagnosis from a clinical standpoint. After the menopause has been thoroughly passed,

---

*A Study of Cancer, p. 8.

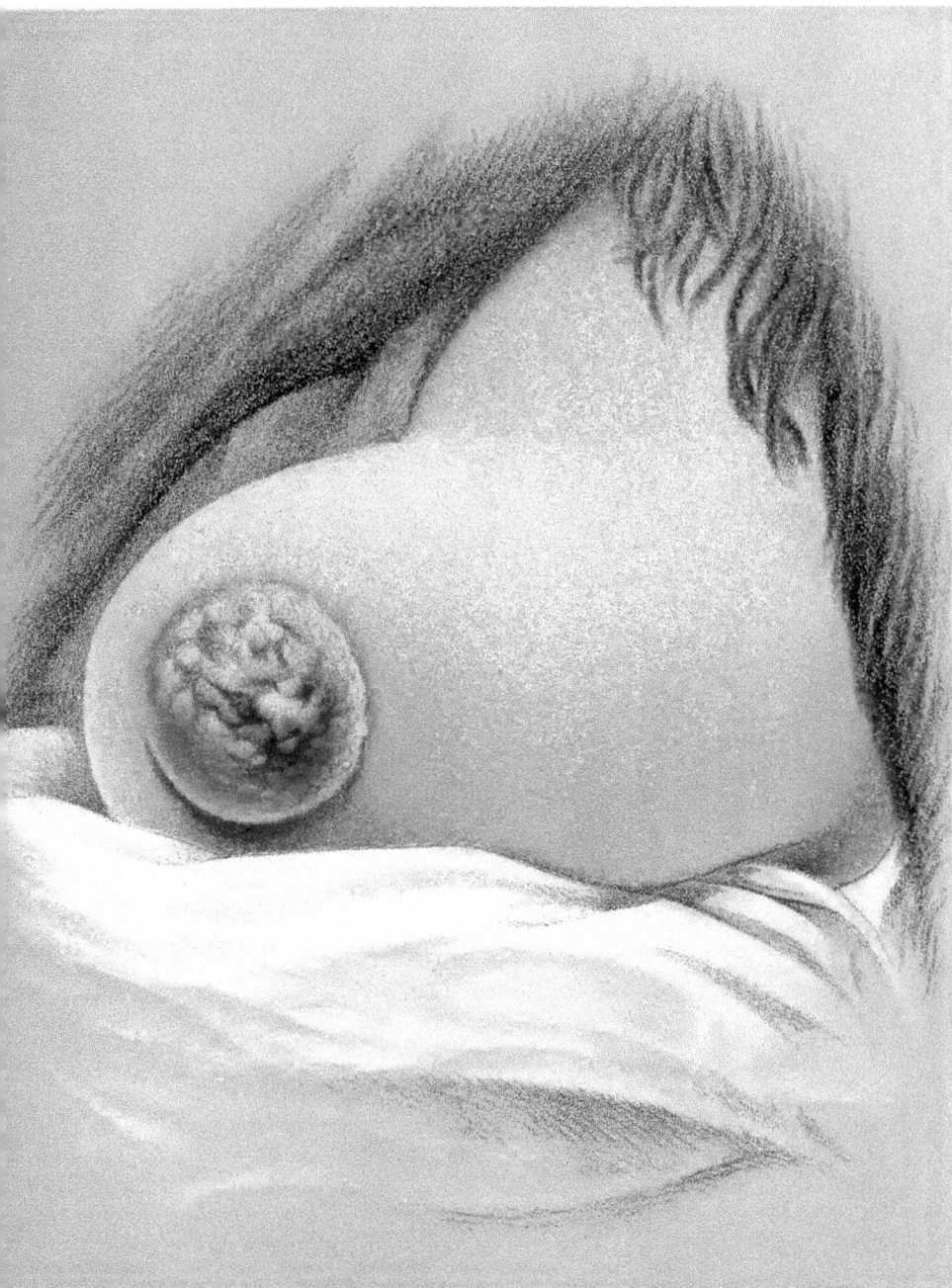

PAGET'S DISEASE OF THE NIPPLE.

every tumor of the breast is probably cancer. In the face of this fact, a patient, 54 years of age, applied to me for treatment with a large scirrhus tumor of the right breast, for which an experienced physician had prescribed an application of tincture of iodine, and expressed the opinion that it was an inflamed milk duct !

The next important step in arriving at a diagnosis is the study of the ætiology of the growth. Has it developed upon any of the pre-cancerous diseases already alluded to ? Is there any history of injury to the part affected, the effects of which have never quite disappeared ? Has there been a history of prolonged local irritation, such as the sharp edge of a tooth against the tongue, for example ? If these questions are answered in the affirmative, the disease is probably cancerous. The question of heredity is of such slight importance that it need only be asked for the purpose of confirming our judgment that it plays a most insignificant part in the causation of cancer.

In the next place, the location of the growth is an important aid in diagnosis. There are several favorite locations for cancer besides the mammary gland. We should look with especial care to disease in the lower lip of a man, or to a scaly patch on the temple, or on the side of the nose, in the neighborhood of the canthus, or on the border of the tongue about midway between the tip and the root.

The symptom of pain is so variable as to be of little aid in diagnosis, even in cancer of the breast, in which cases it is often very slight or entirely absent.

The sense of touch, when educated by experience, is the almost infallible diagnostician of cancer. A man may discard every other means, and yet correctly diagnosticate cancer with his index finger ninety-nine times out of a hundred. It is more unerring than the microscope. This leads me to say of the microscopical examination of malignant growths that its chief value to us as practitioners consists in its invaluable aid to a correct prognosis. It is unnecessary and often impossible to secure a slide for examination until after operation, but *then* it becomes of the greatest interest to know whether the structure of the tumor is of such a nature as to render probable a speedy recurrence or a fatal metastasis. If the microscopist finally succeeds in discovering a cancer bacillus as the real cause of these malignant diseases, he will have added the most important link to the long chain of his valuable discoveries. But we should never be dissuaded from eradicating a suspicious growth because we may have had a section examined which did not show the microscopical characters of carcinoma, sarcoma, or epithelioma. Mr. Butlin* corroborates these views regarding the value of the microscope in the following words:

" It is not always easy to classify a tumor, even

---

* Sarcoma and Carcinoma, p. 9.

though its origin and microscopic structure have been carefully observed. The difference in structure between some adenomas and some carcinomas, between some fibromas or chondromas and some sarcomas, and between the products of some inflammations and some sarcomas, is so very minute, if, indeed, there is a difference, that it is impossible to discover it."

I do not wish to be understood as discrediting in any degree the results or value of microscopical examinations in cancer cases, but to forcibly impress upon the reader the fact that the practitioner must depend upon the clinical features, history, and course of the disease *chiefly*, especially if the early diagnosis of the disease is to be reached and the chances of cure thereby rendered most certain.

I have recently had an interesting experience with a patient for whom we had removed the right breast and axillary contents for carcinoma and, subsequently, six recurrent growths in or near the cicatrix on the chest. At the last operation a small exostosis of the fifth rib was removed (a mistaken procedure, I now believe), and there was great difficulty in healing the wound. After three months, it was decided to remove this stubborn sore, and it was handed to the microscopist, who reported it to be "simple cicatricial tissue." As there was no appearance of any other disease, the axilla having remained free since the first operation three years before, and in view of the fact that the patient's general condition was good, we at once decided that the prognosis was favorable. The sequel proved all our deductions to be incorrect, for in three months there was a large tumor of the spleen, and recurrence also at the very point where this "simple cicatricial tissue" had been found by the microscopist. What other course, then, is to be followed in cases where the diagnosis is uncertain? The question has been partly answered in the preceding chapters, where we advised the removal of all those non-malignant diseases which have been shown to develop into cancer.

All the clinical elements of diagnosis, and the histological characters, should be studied, if possible, and then, if there remains any doubt, *treat it as a cancer.* The question as to whether in this way a breast is sometimes removed which might have been saved must be answered in the affirmative. The removal of a benign tumor, however, is accomplished with such slight risk, and the probability is so great that such a growth will become a source of the fatal chronic irritation of the tissues which produces cancer, that the proper treatment has been employed to give the greatest possible security to the patient. A doubtful or erroneous diagnosis, then, has no disadvantages as far as the patient is concerned in this direction, while to wait for some unmistakable feature of cancer to be manifested, before proceeding to treat it radically, is fraught with extreme danger.

CHAPTER V.

EPITHELIOMA OF THE SKIN—TREATMENT BY MILD CAUTERIZATION—ESCHAROTICS— LACTIC ACID PASTE — JENNINGS' POTASH AND COCAINE PASTE— MARSDEN'S PASTE— BOUGARD'S PASTE.

The most important fact connected with the class of cases under consideration is that ninety per cent. of them are curable if early and efficient treatment be adopted. Cancer in the popular mind has always been regarded as an incurable disease, and yet, according to Marsden's tables,* compiled from the records of over six thousand cases of cancer treated in the London Cancer Hospital, over two thousand, or one-third of the entire number, were surface or epithelial cancer. It is a disease which seldom appears before middle life, when the vital forces are on the decline, and at a period when degeneration of other organs besides the skin is frequently observed. In these cases, then, age is an important factor in ætiology. Reference has already been made to several non-malignant diseases which tend to become cancerous,

---

* A New and Successful Mode of Treating Certain Forms of Cancer, by Alexander Marsden, M. D.

and long continued local irritation is often the exciting cause. Thus an epithelioma finally developed upon the side of the nose in one of my patients at the point where the eye-glasses had rested for many years.

It occurs with far greater frequency in men than in women, Marsden's table making the ratio nearly three to one. Nearly the same proportion is maintained among my own cases. There are certain locations which may be termed the point of election for the disease, by far the greater number being upon the side of the nose, a little before the inner canthus, and upon the temple.

The following description applies to most cases in their early stages.

The patient first notices a small crust, which covers an area of skin perhaps an eighth of an inch in diameter. It is easily removed, but is soon reproduced. After this process has been often repeated, the surface under the scab is found to be raw, and bleeds a little when the crust is first removed. After a variable period, active ulceration begins in the central portion, the borders become slightly elevated and indurated. Then a section through this border will show the usual arrangement of so-called "cell nests" under the microscope, and a disease exists which will never heal unless its most complete destruction is in some way secured. Its course is often slow, and it is not unusual to find a patient who has suffered with an epithelioma of the skin for ten or fifteen years. The rapidity of its course, however, depends, to a large extent, upon the part of the body attacked, being slow if in those parts of the face where there is but little subcutaneous tissue, like the malar region, or upon the scalp, while in the labia majora its course is rapid, and difficult to cure in consequence. Another cause of rapid development is the injudicious employment of comparatively mild caustics.

By the term mild cauterization I mean all caustic applications of whatever kind which aim at a *gradual* destruction of the diseased tissue. A few cases will illustrate my meaning. A young man of thirty years consulted a physician about one year ago for a "cracked" lip, which had troubled him two or three months. During the next six months eighty applications were made to the lip, so the patient says, of a caustic answering to the description of nitrate of silver. The result is the entire lower lip cancerous, an enormous tumor on the left side of the face and inferior maxillary region, which has ulcerated in several places, and the "cancer cachexia" of the older writers indicates an early fatal termination. This very unusual glandular infection can only be accounted for by the fact, as I believe, that the repeated applications acted in the same manner as the local irritation which is so often the exciting cause of the primary disease.

Nitrate of silver is one of the most frequent of

mild applications and also one of the most injurious. It is probable that no epithelioma of the tongue ever escaped an application of this remedy, and it is equally certain that no case was ever benefited thereby.

Pyrogallol and resorcin, both of which have been highly recommended by Unna and others, have been extensively employed, and, as far as my observation of many cases is concerned, I have no hesitation in saying they should never be employed in the treatment of epithelioma of the skin.

It may be stated that no method of treatment should be applied which aims at anything short of complete destruction and removal of all diseased tissue. The only possible exceptions to this rule are occasional instances in which a tongue may be removed to allow of increased facility in feeding; a tumor near the eye, where the sight may be preserved for a time after the one eye has been destroyed, or where a pendulous or ulcerating tumor (as of the breast) may be rendered less painful or offensive for the time being by the removal of a portion of it. Such are palliative measures which may be justifiable, although life is not usually even prolonged thereby.

Cutaneous cancer is usually treated more satisfactorily by escharotics than by any other method, and for various reasons. The patients are usually past middle age, often far advanced in years, and as a class not good subjects for etherization. The antipathy to a surgical operation often leads them to delay treatment until the pre-cancerous stage, as Mr. Jonathan Hutchinson has termed it, has been followed by active malignant characteristics. You can always quite readily persuade them to have a plaster applied. The disease can be thoroughly destroyed by the caustic plasters, for they will all act sufficiently upon diseased tissue in so much less time than upon healthy skin that there is almost an excuse for the fallacy that they exercise a positive power of selection. The resulting cicatrix, when the deep subcutaneous tissues are not involved, is a very smooth, white, and in every way healthy one, far less conspicuous than after removal by operation. Recurrence is no more frequent than after operation, but experience has convinced me that the claim of the cancer quacks that recurrence after caustic is *less* frequent than after removal by the knife is positively groundless. The only cases in which an operation should be preferred to a caustic are those involving the mucous surface of the lip, the eyelids, and all others which have involved a large surface, so that dangerous poisoning might result from absorption.

The choice of a proper escharotic is of considerble importance. If the disease be a very small warty growth, the potassa and cocaine paste of Mr. Jennings is a good one.* The formula is as follows:

---

*Cancer and its Complications, Chas. Egerton Jennings, F. R. C. S., p. 66.

Jennings' Paste.

℞ Cocaine hydrochlorat.............. 2.
    Potass. caustici.................. 12.
    Ung. petrolat. ...   6.
M.

After cleansing the surface and applying a solution of cocaine, this paste is to be rubbed into the growth with a small wooden spatula.

Acetic acid must be at hand to limit its action as soon as desired. Where the disease is that form of epithelioma called rodent ulcer by some, and Jacob's ulcer by other authors, with little or no induration of the borders, a paste composed of lactic acid and salicic acid, in such proportion as to make a thick paste, is effectual in destroying the diseased surface. It has one advantage over others, in that it is not poisonous, and can be spread over a large surface. It is less active than the others, and requires frequent repetition. I now very seldom employ it. The actual cautery is too painful, and patients are much frightened by the very appearance of the doctor armed with a red-hot instrument.

In 1874, in a paper read before the Medical Society of the County of New York, I described the method, then new, of applying an arsenical paste as recommended by Dr. Alexander Marsden, Surgeon-in-Chief of the London Cancer Hospital, and gave histories of twelve cases successfully treated by it. Since that time I have employed the same paste in over one hundred cases. It is satisfactory in the main, and has become a well-recognized remedy throughout this country. In some cases the reaction is very great and the pain very severe, although less is experienced if cocaine is mixed with it.

Marsden's Paste.

℞ Acid arsenioni........................ 4.
   Pulv. acaciæ........................ 2.
M.

This is to be made into a paste *too thick to run*, by very carefully adding cold water, or instead of the powdered acacia, the mucilage may be employed.

It is then applied to only one square inch of the ulcer, covered with cotton to absorb any superfluous paste, and left on until swelling occurs around it with heat and redness, when it is removed, and a line of demarcation usually surrounds the surface cauterized. From one to three days are required to produce the desired effect. Warm poultices are then applied until the slough separates (usually about a week), when, if the disease is all removed, the healing process proceeds as in an ordinary granulating sore. The same process is to be repeated until the disease is all removed. Marsden insists that no cancer of more than four square inches in extent should be thus treated, and only one square inch at a time, and the case very carefully watched. The surgeons of the London Hospital inform me that even Marsden himself seldom employs the paste at present. They have substituted an application called Bougard's paste, after the Belgian surgeon, who first published the formula in his work on caustics.* The author brought it forward as a cure for mammary cancer, but as such, in my judgment, it is open to the same objection as all other caustics; but in cutaneous and lip cases, in fact in all surface epitheliomata where any escharotic is admissible, this is by all odds the best we have at present. It is less painful than Marsden's, forms a more dry and friable slough, can be safely applied to a larger surface, and can always be prepared and ready for instant use, for in a covered jar it will keep for many months. With both pastes the surface must be denuded, if necessary, by caustic potash to render the action prompt and effective in the shortest possible time.

Bougard's formula is as follows:

Wheat flour.............................. 60.
Starch................................... 60.
Arsenic.................................. 1.
Cinnabar................................ 5.
Sal-ammonia .... 5.
Corrosive sublimate.................... 0.50
Solution of chloride of zinc at 52°..... 245.

The first six substances are separately ground and reduced to fine powder. They are then mixed in a mortar of glass or china, and the solution of chlor-

---

* Études sur le Cancer (Brussels, 1882).

ide of zinc is slowly poured in, while the contents are kept rapidly moved with the pestle so that no lumps shall be formed. A thick layer of this is spread on cotton and left in position twenty-four hours, and then managed in every way as Marsden's paste. Few cases require a second application. The ulcer may be dressed with balsam of Peru ointment of varying strengths, according to the stimulation required, and all exuberant granulations are to be kept in check by the usual methods.

An excellent dressing, instead of the Peruvian balsam, is a five or ten-per-cent. aristol ointment, with vaseline as a base. However, this after-treatment is not of vital importance, except in one respect, viz.: *healing under a scab in cancer cases can never be trusted.*

CHAPTER VI.

EPITHELIOMA OF THE EYELIDS AND OF THE LOWER LIP — TREATMENT BY CAUSTICS AND BY OPERATION—EPITHELIOMA OF THE TONGUE—KOCHER'S AND WHITEHEAD'S OPERATIONS— PROGNOSIS ALWAYS UN- FAVORABLE.

Epithelioma of the eyelid finally involves, in a large proportion of cases, the eye itself. The disease usually attacks the lower lid, and a warty growth is frequently the first manifestation. Two years ago a patient now under treatment first noticed en- largement of a small congenital wart on the right lower lid, a little outside of the middle. She squeezed it between the thumb and finger, and some bloody fluid escaped, but no pus. The growth then slightly ulcerated, and very gradually an induration has crept along the outer border of the lid until now it has reached the canthus, and the thickening ex- tends into the body of the lid nearly an eighth of an inch. Some pressure upon the eyeball has resulted, and the conjunctiva is streaked with congested ves- sels, but is apparently free from malignant infection. The usual mistake of calling the disease lupus was repeated in this case, and the repeated application of nitrate of silver has stimulated the growth considerably. I doubt whether the disease began as lupus, but it may have done so. I have seen that transformation occur, but a microscopical section of the growth now shows all the characters of epithelial cancer. The treatment of this particular case will spare the eye, so long as it appears to be healthy. The diseased portion will be excised by scissors, the patient being etherized. Then the gap in the lid will be filled by a flap from the neighborhood, the parts all being carefully secured in position with horse-hair sutures, and the incision painted with aristol collodion (1—30). The eye will then be securely bandaged, and the dressing left undisturbed several days, unless there should be some local or constitutional symptoms referable to the field of operation. This typical case is here given, with the treatment, to emphasize the fact that all cancer of the eyelid, whether of small extent or of the most serious character, should be removed at once, and only by operation. Caustics of every description are contraindicated in this region, for they are not only inefficient, but positively harmful. During the past three weeks I have extirpated the eye for two patients, removing the entire upper and lower lids in both cases, for epithelioma which has been treated over two years' with the utmost thoroughness, by curetting and caustics of various kinds, but the progress of the malady has scarcely been impeded thereby, and the eyesight in each case has been nearly destroyed. It should be stated that, when not more than one-third óf the border of the lid is involved, it can often be successfully removed by cutting away an elliptical piece without a plastic operation, as it will heal kindly by granulation. In case undue pressure is caused by the cicatrix, a simple canthoplasty will relieve it.

One word more regarding extirpation for cancer. It is not a dangerous operation, and it is frequently successful in effecting a permanent cure. All the contents of the orbit should be removed with curved scissors, and the cavity then closely packed with moist aristol gauze and tightly bandaged, to prevent hæmorrhage. It is likely to be a bloody operation, but it is difficult to take up the vessels, so I hasten through the operation and apply the dressings as quickly as possible. Several patients have had no recurrence after this operation, although performed from five to seven years ago. Their ages ranged from sixty to eighty-one years.

EPITHELIOMA OF THE LOWER LIP.

Nearly twelve per cent. of my cases have been cancer of the lower lip, and all were men, with one exception. The oldest patient was eighty-two and the youngest twenty-six, the average age being fifty-five, so that the disease is pre-eminently one of old age. Only twenty-one per cent. were smokers, so that the use of the pipe plays a small part in the ætiology. Any ulcer, fissure, or scab on the lower lip of an old man is probably cancerous if it persists for any length of time, especially when resisting treatment by ordinary remedies. Fortunately, nearly all begin in or near the median line and outside of the lip. For that reason, when the disease is small, it may be best treated with caustics, Bougard's paste being the most satisfactory. Its action is prompt, twenty-four hours sufficing to destroy the growth, and under poultices, applied in a muslin pouch, held in position by tapes tied around the neck, the slough will separate in about four days, the resulting cicatrix being imperceptible. The plaster is held in position by collodion and the patient cautioned against touching it with the tongue, for fear of poisoning. *The case should be carefully watched while the paste is on the lip.*

When the cancer has attacked the entire thickness of the lip, and has passed below the vermilion border, excision is the only remedy. Any projecting tooth should be removed, and, with the lip firmly held on both sides by the thumb and finger of an assistant, a free removal is made by two curved incisions, thus: U instead of the usual V incision, which has always been recommended. The advantage of the curved incision consists in a more even distribution of the traction caused by the sutures, and the occasional difficulty of securing perfect union at the border after the V incision is thereby, avoided. The edges are adjusted and stitched with interrupted horse-hair sutures, the incision being then well painted with the aristol collodion and left undisturbed until union is complete. I seldom apply a bandage or any other dressing, simply cautioning the patient against opening the mouth or in any way stretching the tissues of the lip. The prognosis is excellent in these cases, unless treatment is delayed, in which case it becomes exceedingly grave, especially if the angle of the mouth is involved, or the cervical glands affected. Early diagnosis and prompt removal mean success, while the reverse invites probable failure.

EPITHELIOMA OF THE TONGUE.

I have never seen a cancer of the tongue of any but the epithelial type. At the same time it is true that a sarcoma is very rarely found here, such as Dr. Jacobi's case, in an infant the day after birth, which was removed and examined with the microscope a couple of months afterwards.* The mere fact that a disease of the tongue of a cancerous character appears very rarely in a young person under thirty renders it probable that the disease is epithelioma, if the patient has passed that age. There is no question of the correctness of the rule that sarcoma is a disease of early life, and that epithelioma and carcinoma belong to the later period, but there are occasional exceptions in both cases.

The tongue is not only subject to epithelial cancer, but in the frequency with which it suffers there-

---

* American Journal of Obstetrics, 1870.

from it has but one rival, that being the uterus. Mr. Jessett has analyzed 2,227 cases, occurring in the London Cancer Hospital during the ten years ending in 1881, of which 8.5 per cent. were the tongue, 12.3 per cent. in the uterus, and 31.3 per cent. in the female breast. From my 534 cases it appears that 6.3 per cent. were in the tongue, 4.3 per cent. in the uterus, and 26.5 per cent. in the mamma. There is an evident explanation of the difference between my percentages and Mr. Jessett's, Mr. Henry Morris', Sir James Paget's, and others, which shows how misleading individual statistics may be, in fact *usually are*, in regard to frequency of diseases of special organs. This explanation is the fact that patients apply to specialists for advice, and thus it happens that the gynæcologist finds a great preponderance of cancer in the uterus, almost none of the tongue, and comparatively few of the breast, because tumor cases occurring in the breast drift to the general surgeon. Those of us who are connected with the New York Skin and Cancer Hospital see an undue proportion of epithelioma of the skin. Jessett's tables, made up from the general records of the Cancer Hospital, are more nearly correct in regard to this point than any individual case records.

Cancer of the tongue, like epithelioma of the lip, is a disease of men, the exceptions being very few, only three of my thirty-four cases being women. At the risk of repeating to some extent what has already

been said regarding ætiology, the following table of
causes may be profitably considered:

Predisposing Causes....
{
Age.
Sex.
Leucoma.
Psoriasis.
Ichthyosis,
Syphilis.
Spirit-drinking.
Smoking.
Rough eating.
}

Exciting Causes ....
{
Caustics.
Bad teeth.
Dental plates.
Irritation of pipe.
Salivary calculi.
}

Syphilis plays an important part among the predisposing causes of cancer of the tongue. Its influence, however, is an indirect one. A gumma appears
on the tongue, or a fissure, or a simple ulcer. It is
frequently cauterized with a mild caustic—nitrate of
silver, sulphate of copper, or some similar application—but a cure is not effected. The habits of spirit-
drinking, smoking and chewing of tobacco, and the
use of irritating food, all combine to keep up a
chronic irritation of the sore, and thus is developed a
cancerous degeneration of the epithelium.

It should be carefully noted that nearly all the
causes named, both predisposing and exciting, are of
a character to be successfully treated or avoided if the
physician has a just appreciation of their relation to
the development of cancer. The average age of my

cases, when the disease was first discovered, was fifty-two years, so that when a man of that age, or older, presents himself with an ulcer of the tongue, it should be considered as a pre-cancerous disease at least, if it has not already passed across the line into the region of incurable disease.

TREATMENT.

The extreme difficulty in the way of successful treatment depends upon the histological character of the tongue. An organ of spongy tissue, with a wealth of blood-vessels and nerves; an organ almost always in motion, and, by its very location, extremely liable to irritation, furnishes an unrivaled soil for the dissemination of the cancer elements far beyond the original seat of the disease. The first requisite for our guidance in instituting a plan of treatment is to treat it *early* and *thoroughly*. While this is true of all cancer, wherever located, it is, if possible, more necessary in cancer of the tongue than in disease of any other organ. As a rule, caustics are not admissible. The pastes of all descriptions are dangerous on account of their deadly ingredients. If extreme care is used, the fused potash or soda may be applied to disease of the tongue in the very earliest stage.

A man, aged thirty-five, who had been syphilitic for several years, developed a warty growth on the left border of the tongue one and a half inches from the tip, upon the site of an old ulcer. It was indurated, somewhat painful, and a renewal of specific treatment failed to reduce it in size, or even to modify its character. It was completely destroyed by caustic potash at one sitting, and after nine years it has not recurred. I believe the growth was malignant. The actual cautery in any form would have been equally efficacious, but is a more formidable agent in the estimation of the patient. Mild cauterization, as I have before remarked, is extremely harmful in cancer of the tongue, and many cases which call for a formidable operation have been stimulated to rapid and destructive growth by these applications. Unfortunately, the disease is usually pretty well advanced before we are consulted in regard to treatment.

Seventeen years ago I first witnessed an amputation of the tongue by Prof. Henry B. Sands. The method employed was the same now employed by Morant Baker, except that the galvanic écraseur was used instead of whipcord. The mouth was well opened, and the attachments to the jaw divided by scissors, passed as near the bone as possible, until the tongue was free some distance beyond the seat of the disease. A strong silk loop was passed through the two tips of the tongue, for traction purposes, and the tongue then incised in the middle of the dorsum, and the two sides separated at the septum down to its root. Then long, blunt needles were passed through on the line of the proposed removal, the loop of the écraseur passed behind the needles, and the first half slowly cut away with the wire, heated only to a red heat. This process is to be repeated for the other half when deemed necessary, which, I am inclined to believe, is always preferable to a partial amputation. This operation is strongly advocated on the ground that it is attended with a considerably smaller mortality than a cutting operation. However, bleeding vessels, if there be any, are not so securely tied after this method of removal as after an ordinary operation, and, while less blood is lost during the removal, secondary hæmorrhage is more likely to follow, and, during the separation of the slough, septic infection is more liable to ensue than when a clean cut is granulating. The importance of thorough and frequent cleansing and disinfecting of the surface now appears to me of vital moment, and it is possible that by doing this the stump can be kept free from suppurative processes, even after the galvano-caustic operation. A battery, even of the most approved make, is sometimes imperfect, and special skill in its management is absolutely essential.

It is usually more desirable to remove the tongue by some of the well known operations, and of these I shall only refer to Kocher's, Billroth's, and Whitehead's methods. Kocher attempts to prevent the somewhat frequent accident of septic pneumonia, by plugging the pharynx with antiseptic gauze after inserting a tracheotomy tube, the patient being fed twice a day when the packing of the pharynx and mouth is removed. Incision is made along the side of the neck into the floor of the mouth, and this is preceded by ligature of the lingual artery in both Kocher's and Billroth's operations. .It is needless to say that the operations are complicated ones and often difficult, and in Kocher's the tracheotomy is an added danger, which counterbalances any immunity from pneumonia which the packing of the pharynx is intended to prevent. The amount of shock is considerably increased by the tracheotomy and ligation of the artery.

Whitehead's operation is far simpler in its details, and, in my experience, quite satisfactory. I have never had a death due to any fault of the method. A good gag (I prefer O'Dwyer's to any other), a pair of curved scissors, and some Halstead artery forceps are the only instruments required. After the attachments to the jaw and floor of the mouth are divided and the tongue split, each half is well pulled forward by the traction loops which are held by assistants, and the tongue is snipped off with the scissors, the ranine artery being caught the moment it is divided, or even before. Should there be any difficulty in placing a good ligature, the clamp may be left in place for forty-eight hours, after which the vessel will not bleed. Mr. Christopher Heath's valuable suggestion should never be forgotten, even by the nurse, that hæmorrhage may be controlled by hooking the finger over the root of the stump, and dragging it forward, thus producing firm and efficient pressure.

They tell us that any enlarged glands should be removed *before* the tongue is cut, but I would modify this rule by saying that, if the glands are enlarged, it is not a suitable case for operation of any description. I know of no justifiable operation in case of recurrence of the disease after amputation of the tongue. The after-treatment often determines the success or failure of whatever method of removal has been adopted. The wound should be kept lightly dusted with aristol or iodoform, and for a week at least the patient should be fed artificially by means of a tube passed into the stomach, or by nutritive enemata, or by both, according to the requirements of the case. The mouth should be frequently sprayed by an antiseptic fluid, but no attempt at the use of a gargle or lotion should be made, for the most perfect rest of the stump is necessary for at least one week.

The removal of the tongue for cancer involves some risk under the most favorable circumstances, the mortality ranging from seven to twenty per cent., according to the statistics of various authors. A fair idea of the results of operations in other cases may be gained from Mr. Butlin's table of seventy cases.* Eight died of the operation itself; in nineteen there is no record; thirty-two were dying of recurrence, or

---

* Operative Surgery of Malignant Disease.

dead; in only five cases was there a complete and perfect cure extending beyond the three-year limit.

Several of my thirty-four cases were incurable before they came under my care. Of those treated, the one where caustic potash was used remains well after nine years; one is still under the aniline chloride treatment; one has recurrence in the glands one and a half years after operation, and the others, as far as we are able to complete the history, are dead. I am forced to the conclusion that cancer of the tongue is one of the most deadly of the whole group, and, unless removal is undertaken in the very earliest stage of the malady, the prognosis is most unfavorable, and is never good in any case.

CHAPTER VII.

CANCER OF THE FEMALE BREAST; FREQUENCY, ÆTIOLOGY, AND CLINICAL FEATURES; DIAGNOSIS.

The most frequent form of cancer in the female breast is scirrhus carcinoma. In Satterthwaite and Porter's table of one hundred unselected cases of cancer, forty-one belonged to this class. In the 10,759 cases reported by Marsden, 5,706 were scirrhus—more than one-half. In my own table of 534 cases, 139 were in the female breast, and of these 89 were scirrhus. We properly assume, therefore, that this variety of cancer is typical, while the various other forms are more or less widely divergent modifications of scirrhus. The term "cancer of the female breast" is considered more comprehensive than "cancer of the mammary gland," because all cancer of the breast does not belong to the mammary gland *primarily*, but invades the gland by the usual methods of extension which, in breast cancer, according to Mr. Bryant,* are as follows:

"1. By continuous local infection, or other gradual involvement of surrounding structures, in the order of their arrangement around the primary seat of the disease; by progressive infiltration, as well as

---

* Diseases of the Breast.

by extension along the perivascular sheaths of the blood-vessels of the diseased part, this being a common feature of scirrhus.

" 2. By lymphatic infection, by which is meant the infiltration of the lymphatic glands associated with the primary diseased centre, or its coverings; by the lymphatic ducts, which carry the cancer elements to the glands by the lymph, or the ducts themselves become directly infiltrated.

" 3. Secondary or vascular infection, by which is meant the propagation of the disease through the blood currents. By this method probably multiple secondary growths, similar to the primary disease, are found in the viscera or other parts of the body, often remote from the primary seat of the disease."

I must be permitted to take exception to Mr. Bryant's unqualified statement that in carcinoma of the breast the gland structure is the one *primarily* involved. If that were absolutely true, Dr. S. W. Gross' title of "cancer of the mammary gland" would be the more correct one. The cancer following eczema of the nipple primarily involved the skin and secondarily invaded the mammary gland. Undoubtedly the vast majority of cases originate in the gland itself, but there are many exceptions to the rule.

A patient, fifty-nine years old, applied for treatment February 21, 1889, with a large scirrhus tumor of the left breast, which had invaded the axilla and encircled the axillary vein in its growth. It began four years before as a small tubercle in the *skin*, about half an inch above and outside of the nipple.

Another patient, aged fifty-two, was treated by operation March 3, 1890, whose disease (scirrhus) began in a fissure of the nipple which had not healed since the last child was nursed, eight years before. From this point the entire mammary gland had become infiltrated with cancer.

Mrs. M. K., aged thirty-eight, was operated upon June 25, 1887, for the removal of a scirrhus carcinoma of the left breast, which began in a *wart on the skin near the nipple*. Several other cases are recorded in my note-book, where cancer of the breast did not originate in the mammary gland, but the above histories are sufficient to show that Mr. Bryant's statement should have been somewhat less positive.

ÆTIOLOGY OF CANCER OF THE BREAST.

Some points in regard to the cause of cancer of the breast are of such importance that I wish to briefly consider them, even at the risk of repeating what has been said in a previous chapter. As in cancer of the lip, and of various other parts of the body, a prolonged irritation is sufficient to produce malignant disease, so in breast cancer we find this fact frequently emphasized. A striking example of this is the final development of cancer of the female breast beginning in the remains of an old mammary abscess, occurring five, ten, and even twenty years before.

The patient will tell you that there was always a little lump there, and the soreness remaining after the ab scess was cured had never entirely disappeared. The cancerous disease began when the patient reached that time in life when such degeneration usually occurs. Traumatism is an important factor in the æti- ology of this class. In my 139 cases, twenty-three gave a reliable history of a blow, or some other injury, with which she connected the development of the tumor, and in most instances, I have no doubt, the patient was correct. In one instance a watch had been carried in the bosom for many years, resting upon the same portion of the breast year after year, until a slight tenderness and pain were noticed, which gradually increased until the watch was removed and the breast examined, when I found a small tumor, which was removed, and by microscopical examination proved to be cancer.

The fact is that a study of the causes producing these neoplasms of the female breast indicates, be- yond reasonable doubt, that the so-called " local " origin of cancer, as opposed to the theory of a " con- stitutional " cause, is correct. It would seem to be unnecessary to argue in favor of the local theory after the discussion of the subject in the London Pathological Society in 1874, which Mr. Jennings* has recently reviewed, were it not for the fact

---

* Cancer and Its Complications. 1889.

that many doctors and patients continue to regard cancer as a "blood disease," and consequently incurable by operative procedures. The evidence in favor of the purely local origin of cancer is now so generally credited by those who have studied carefully the natural history of the disease, that Sir James Paget stands *almost* alone in his advocacy of the "constitutional" theory. Several times during the past few years we have been upon the very threshold of the discovery of the cancer bacillus, and when it is found, as it doubtless will be, the last support of the "constitutional" or "blood origin" hypothesis will be swept away. Permit me here to quote Mr. Jennings' conclusion in full upon this point:

"1. Cancer first affects the body locally, spreads locally, and invades the body along definite tracks (lymphatic and vascular systems).

"2. Cancer grows plant-like in a congenial soil.

"3. Some soils are more congenial than others to the development of cancer (predisposition), and tissues peculiarly favorable to the propagation of cancer, or the reverse, may be acquired by inheritance.

"4. The disease can be completely eradicated by surgical operations; and, when they fail, the inference is that they had not been undertaken sufficiently early nor with sufficient boldness."

CLINICAL FEATURES.

The following history of a case, which was under my care from the very commencement to its fatal termination, and in which the patient persistently refused all treatment until it was too late to secure even a palliation of symptoms by operation, furnishes an excellent description of the clinical features of the disease: Mrs. R., age 62, widow, the mother of several children, had always been healthy until one year ago, when she fell from a chair and received a contusion of the right breast, which, it should be stated, was large and pendulous. It was painful and very tender for a few days, after which a small, sharply circumscribed portion only attracted her attention if pressed upon by the clothing or otherwise. After six months this point began to increase in size, a slight enlargement of the breast was observed, which steadily increased from that time, until at the end of eighteen months the entire mammary gland was of a stony hardness, darting pains were frequent in the breast and along the course of the lymphatics into the axilla, along the arm, and even down the forearm. At this time some of the axillary glands were enlarged. The tumor became less movable on the chest wall, and from the nipple, which had become retracted, a few drops of serosanguinolent fluid occasionally exuded. The skin over the tumor became gradually livid on the most prominent portion, the tumor began to soften, finally ulcerated, and a fungoid growth sprang up, which in turn broke down, and the open sore steadily became larger and deeper, until the thin and offensive discharges kept the clothing saturated, nothwithstanding the utmost care on the part of the attendants. This was two years from the beginning of the disease, and then appeared the general constitutional symptoms. A large tumor of the supra-clavicular gland of that side appeared, and the patient lost appetite, strength, and flesh. Loss of sleep and occasional hæmorrhages (not profuse) carried her rapidly along the downward road, until the end of the third year, when she died. For three months the entire upper extremity had been œdematous and utterly useless. There was no history of heredity, and her knowledge of the family was unusually complete. This record, with a few minor changes due to age, differences of temperament, and variety in the exciting cause, would represent the symptoms and course of the vast majority of cases of cancer of the female breast. In a younger patient its course would probably have been shorter; in an older one it might have been prolonged much beyond three years. Dr. John T. Kennedy, of New York City, has recently informed me of an undoubted case of cancer of the breast of seventeen years' duration, and the patient is still in good general health.

I have had only one other case which followed its natural course, and that patient lived seven years, and the constitutional infection did not occur until

5 DDD

the last year of life. Both of these tumors were carcinoma, and my experience has not demonstrated the correctness of the opinion held by some writers, that traumatism is more often followed by sarcoma than by any other form of cancer.

It is desirable to make an accurate diagnosis in all cases of tumor of the female breast, yet I repeat that non-malignant neoplasms in this organ are undoubtedly so frequently the precancerous stage of the disease that we should not insist upon a positive diagnosis before deciding to remove the growth.

By a careful study we may usually classify these tumors, and make the differential diagnosis sufficiently early to insure the success of operative treatment. I have found such satisfaction in the rules laid down by Dr. S. W. Gross* that I am certain we cannot find a more complete statement of the subject than can be gained by a review of his conclusions. The first rule he lays down should not be neglected, viz.: Both breasts should be fully exposed for purposes of comparison, and the patient be placed in a recumbent posture. By this means the resistance of the chest wall enables us to detect any nodule, however small, which might escape detection if the gland is simply pinched up between the thumb and finger, while the

* Tumors of the Mammary Gland, Chapter xi.

patient is sitting or standing. The great advantage of this mode of examination has been demonstrated in my own practice frequently.

Gross has compared carcinomatous with non-carcinomatous tumors, and included the sarcomas in the latter class, a distinction which I believe is often misleading, and the term *cancerous* tumor is better for clinical purposes. Inasmuch as his cases of carcinoma outnumber all others in the proportion of more than 5 to 1, we may make safe deductions therefrom.

AGE OF DEVELOPMENT.

The average age of cancer patients is forty-eight years, and it never develops before the twentieth year —77.26 per cent. develop after the age of forty. In impubic girls the idea of cancer may be discarded.

HEREDITARY PREDISPOSITION.

Cancer is traceable to heredity in 11.28 per cent. of all cases, while non-cancerous tumors do not appear to be inherited.

SITUATION.

Most common at upper and *outer* margin, and not infrequent near the nipple. The non-cancerous growths usually at the upper and *inner* circumference, rarely near the nipple.

CONSISTENCE.

Uniformly densely hard and inelastic throughout, except in rare instances of combination with an involution cyst, when there is a limited spot of fluctuation. As an exception, may be firm and elastic, or even soft and fluctuating.

MULTIPLICITY.

Several tumors are rarely present in the same breast.

MOBILITY.

Move with the gland of which they form a part, and cannot be isolated. Attachments to the skin and chest are common, and frequently extensive. Non-cancerous tumors glide and roll under the fingers, and move freely within the mamma and on the adjacent parts.

STATE OF THE NIPPLE.

The nipple is permanently retracted and fixed in 52 per cent. of all cases, and is often infiltrated. A thin, sanguinolent discharge is met with in 9 per cent. of all cases, but it is never copious.

CONDITION OF THE SKIN.

The skin, even when the tumor is not larger than a hazel-nut, provided it be superficial, is dimpled and adherent. In larger growths it is adherent, thinned, or discolored, or rigid and brawny from specific infiltration in 34.54 per cent. of all cases, and the seat of distinct nodules in 10.61 per cent. In other tumors it is never dimpled nor the seat of secondary tubers.

LYMPHATIC GLANDS.

The axillary glands are enlarged and hard when the patient first comes under observation in 64.23 per cent. of all cases, and in one out of every 22 instances the glands of the neck are also involved. In other tumors the axillary glands are enlarged in only 2.98 per cent. of all examples, and the supra-clavicular glands are never implicated.

Under the above headings I have given Prof. Gross' percentages, but they correspond with my own to a remarkable degree. While I have copied his own words for the most part, I have given only the points of greatest value, and they are sufficient to render a diagnosis of cancer of the breast easy and certain in a vast majority of cases.

CHAPTER VIII.

CANCER OF THE FEMALE BREAST (CONTINUED) — TREATMENT — CAUSTIC TREATMENT NEVER TO BE RECOMMENDED—OPERA- TION —- DETAILS OF OPERATION— DRESSINGS— RESULTS— CAN- CER OF THE MALE BREAST.

TREATMENT.

Many elaborate plans have been formulated and recommended, looking to the removal of cancer of the breast by caustic applications. While these differ one from the other in the agent employed, or in the methods of using them, the effects are substantially the same, namely, the production of a slough in the diseased tissue and its surroundings, leaving a deep irregular ulcer to be healed by granulation.

It is not necessary, for my purpose, to review all the different methods, but I will give a single instance of the use of Marsden's paste, in a cancer of the breast, which came under my notice.

Mrs. B., aged 55, who, thirty years previously, had an epithelioma of the nose successfully treated by a caustic, developed a scirrhous tumor of the left breast, which involved a considerable portion of the gland, although there was no disease of the axillary glands. It was as good a case for the use of caustics as we ever find in the breast, and Marsden's paste was applied by the attending physician, according to the rules which have been given in a previous chapter. In due time a large slough separated, but it was evident that the deeper portion of the ulcer was still cancerous. The paste was re-applied to this portion, which was in the lower part. of the excavation and about three-quarters of an inch below the surface. There was considerable secretion from the ulcer at the time of the application, and as the patient was lying in bed, some of this purulent matter collected in the groove where the paste was applied, kept it somewhat softened, and its caustic effect was not satisfactory. The natural sequence was the absorption of the poison, and a general paralysis occurred, affecting all the extremities, and rendering the patient permanently helpless. At this juncture I saw the case for the first time, and removed the entire cicatrix by operation. The healing was satisfactory, and although the patient lived eight years afterwards, there was no recurrence of cancer. The immediate cause of death was some acute affection, but the arsenical paralysis continued to the last. All will agree that in this instance caustic treatment was a failure, and it is my judgment, after repeated observations of such treatment, that no case of cancer of the breast can be as successfully managed by caustics as by operation, and it is my habit to advise patients to avoid their use, as such treatment is tedious, painful, ineffectual in most instances, and often dangerous.

Even Bougard's paste, which I have so highly recommended in the treatment of cancer of the skin, is open
to the same objections as all other caustics, and should
also be discarded in breast cases.

The operation for removal of a cancerous breast
is comparatively simple, especially when the disease
is limited to the mammary gland.   If the axillary or
subclavicular lymphatic glands have been invaded, or
in cases where the skin is extensively diseased, the
operation is often both formidable and difficult.

Two important points in regard to the operation
are still under discussion by surgeons.   The first
refers to the advisability of opening the axilla when
the glands are not the seat of disease.   The answer
should be positively in favor of doing so, when we
consider the incontrovertible fact that recurrence
occurs in these glands in a *very large* proportion of
cases.   It is but common sense to declare that, if the
glands are removed, one great danger of recurrence
is thereby avoided.   It is also true that we are never
able to decide with certainty that the axillary contents are free from infection until we have exposed
them to view.   In one instance it was the opinion
of my assistants, as well as my own, that the lymphatics were healthy *before* the incision was made, but
afterwards the entire chain of glands, from the breast
to the axillary space, and under the pectoral muscles

as well, were found to be cancerous, and twenty-seven glands, with all the cellular tissue surrounding them, were removed. It should be noted that the operation was nine years ago, and the patient is still living and has never had a recurrence. The disease was scirrhus carcinoma.

If we leave the axillary contents undisturbed, a recurrence of the disease is not only to be feared, but is actually rendered probable. It is almost as reprehensible surgical practice as to leave a portion of the mammary gland when the tumor happens to be small, a proceeding which no one of mature judgment now considers for a moment. We are told that to remove the contents of the axilla considerably increases the dangers of the operation. My own experience does not sustain that opinion. Although I have made it an invariable rule for many years to open the axilla, I have yet to see any serious consequences therefrom, and the extremely small death rate from the operation has not been increased. The danger from amputation of the breast is not to be considered for a moment when compared with the risk of recurrence of the disease, and I repeat that this is vastly diminished by opening the axilla.

The other mooted question has been prominently brought forward by Dr. S. W. Gross, who carried our argument in favor of the axillary operation (which he advocated) still further, and advised the removal of a very large section of the skin over and around the breast, leaving an extensive wound to heal by granulation. He recommended removal of the breast by a circular incision, which would include all the mammary gland and its coverings, together with all paramammary tissues, fascia, adipose tissue, and muscle, and, of course, making it impossible to leave any flaps which could be brought together. In some extreme cases this procedure is a necessity, but to make such an operation the rule in all cases is unwise. In the tedious process of healing such a large surface by granulation, with the resulting extensive cicatrix, a new cause of recurrence is encountered. This is especially the case if the cicatricial tissue develops a tendency to contract, as is frequently the case. The safer course lies in *prompt, rapid,* and *complete* union of cutaneous surfaces, such as can always be secured if an early diagnosis and immediate removal are effected. The advantages of this course are so evident that I have been enabled to make the prognosis with certainty by noting whether we have a rapid or tardy reparative process after the operation.

DETAILS OF THE OPERATION.

The special preparation of the patient for the operation of removal of the breast and the axillary contents consists in cleansing and shaving the skin of the axilla, and thoroughly rubbing into the entire field of operation a one-per-cent. solution of carbolic acid in pure olive oil, as recommended by Mr. Nunn.*

---

* Nunn on Cancer of the Breast.

This should be done on the day preceding the operation. All antiseptic precautions should be thoroughly observed, for we aim to secure primary union of the axillary incision and as much of the remaining cut as possible.

The patient is placed squarely upon the back and an assistant holds the arm steadily at *right angles with the trunk*, and not above that point, as some suggest, for by that means the axillary vessels are drawn out of their natural relations, and thus possibly confuse the operator. The amount of tissue to be included in the elliptical incisions is to be determined *entirely* by the extent of the tumor, ample distance being allowed for an extension of the infiltration beyond the line of evident disease. The general direction of the incisions should nearly correspond with the fibres of the great pectoral muscle, as the best drainage is thereby secured while the patient is in a recumbent posture. Then with a sharp scalpel, so held that the plane of the blade is vertical to the skin, which is held taut by the thumb and fingers of the left hand, by a single sweep the first incision is carried from a point near the sternum under the breast to a point on a vertical line from the axilla. If possible, cut all adipose and connective tissue to the fascia by this first stroke. Clamp any vessels large enough to require it, and make the opposite upper incision to meet the two extremities of the first one. Then, grasping the included mass with the left hand, it is rapidly detached down to the muscles beneath and removed. While Mr. Stile's method of detecting whether the incisions have been through diseased tissue by treating the part removed with dilute nitric acid, which turns the cancerous tissue white, is an ingenious one, it should be unnecessary, for we at once proceed to remove *all* cellular tissue left in the floor of the wound, then the fascia, and finally the muscle itself, *in every instance.* All vessels which have been secured by the forceps are then tied, and the cavity filled with a towel wrung dry from very hot carbolized or bi-chloride water, taking care before doing so to loosen the flaps well to facilitate bringing them together afterwards. The incision for the axillary operation is then carried from the outer angle of the wound along the border of pectoralis major entirely beyond the axilla, and then the dissection must be carefully made with the handle of the knife and the fingers until the axillary vein is reached, which must be the starting point of all satisfactory work in these cases. Then by working downward, using the blade of the instrument or scissors but seldom (after the flaps have been well turned back), the remaining removal is very easy. If the tumor is found to have involved the axillary vessels, we have a complication of grave import, and in such cases *recurrence is certain,* ·no matter what course we take regarding it. I believe it is just as well to close the wound after removing what lies below the vessels as to undertake the difficult task of ferreting out disease which has implicated the vessels and invaded the space beyond them. The next step consists in examining underneath the pectoral muscles and removing all glands there found as far as the lower border of the clavicle, using the fingers alone in this search. Cut the muscles away, if they are diseased, without the slightest hesitation, as the patient may have very good use of the shoulder without them.

After ligating the vessels, fill this cavity with a hot towel also, and proceed to close the first wound, by a continuous horse-hair suture, beginning at the sternal end. If the flaps are too short in some places to unite, bring them as near together as possible, and afterwards relieve tension upon them by fastening strips of gauze an inch and a half wide and eight inches or more in length to the skin above and below with collodion, and then tie the opposite ends securely together. This is a suggestion of Bougard's which I have found valuable in many cases. Then paint the sutured line with aristol collodion (1.–30.). Beginning at the outer end, close the axillary incision in the same manner, placing a little bundle of horse-hair in the cavity for drainage. It is seldom necessary to place any drainage in the first or mammary wound. In fact, a drainage tube here often delays repair. A layer of moist aristol gauze is then laid over the entire wound, and this in turn, and the well breast, covered with a thick layer of cotton, and a six-inch gauze bandage firmly applied. The bandage should finally inclose the arm, but the forearm should be left free, and placed in an ordinary sling. Then it can be occasionally straightened, and in this way the entire limb is rendered more comfortable, and a better circulation therein secured.

It may be stated here that my reason for preferring horse-hair to any other suture is that by simple washing it can be made perfectly aseptic, and it can be left in position indefinitely, without the slightest irritation or suppuration, and it is as indestructible as silver wire. If the hair is wet, it becomes as pliable as catgut, and can be as securely fastened by the ordinary knot.

For several reasons I prefer the continuous suture, and a little device suggested to me by Dr. J. F. Aitken in regard to fastening the ends is valuable. It consists in leaving a long end to the hair as last brought out, and running a loop through the opposite flap when the double end and the single one can be easily and firmly tied. The advantage of this little manœuvre will be fully appreciated after you have tried the ordinary ways of making a *single* end fast without allowing the suture to slip.

I never change or disturb the dressing under five or six days unless it becomes moistened by drainage, or some rise in the patient's temperature is noticed, when the dressing should be changed. The subsequent care of the wound is to be determined by circumstances, and requires no special mention. I have been thus minute, and even elementary, in describing the operation simply because regard to these comparatively unimportant details, if neglected even in part, often jeopardizes the success of the operation.

I wish to add a few words regarding the results of the operation. In my cases only two deaths have occurred as the immediate sequence of the operation. One of these was extremely septic at the time we operated, and I suffered from a severe inflammation of one finger, and one assistant had a similar uncomfortable experience. The patient died of peritonitis. The other fatal case was a patient who had been living in a malarial district, and a violent intermittent fever caused death from exhaustion, one week after the operation. Thus we are justified in saying that the danger from the removal of the breast by operation is very slight indeed.

All the patients who had disease in the neighborhood of the axillary vessels have suffered from recurrence, and, as far as their histories can be verified, have died of the disease.

In this class of cases, then, the prognosis is always unfavorable.

In the other cases we can report a number of permanent cures. One is well after fifteen years, one after nine years, another died of a different disease eight years after operation, and twenty are known to have passed the three-year limit and remained well. Several have had slight recurrent growths removed, and are still free from disease and in good health. We have here, then, to repeat what we have so often said regarding cancer in other parts of the body, viz., that if the operation is performed at a very early stage of the disease, success is almost assured; but if treatment is delayed for years, months, or even weeks after the tumor is discovered, it is at the patient's peril, and no surgeon should ever consent to such fatal procrastination.

CANCER OF THE MALE BREAST.

There is no especial interest connected with cancer of the male breast except regarding its frequency.

One case of my 141 occurred in the left breast of a man of 42, who received a blow about a year previously. There was no axillary involvement, and the tumor, which was as large as a goose-egg, was easily removed, and proved to be a spindle-celled sarcoma. He died within a year, of a general sarcomatous disease appearing in the form of over one hundred nodules on the skin all over the body, varying in size from a pea to a walnut. He gave no family history of cancer, and was a splendid specimen of muscular development, even when the operation was performed.

Dr. S. W. Gross has made a *résumé* from different authorities, showing about the same relative frequency as my own:

"Sir James Paget believes that of every 100

cases of cancer of the mamma only 2 occur in men. Of 102 examples of which I (Gross) have a record, I have seen only 2 in males. Billroth, out of 252 cases, had 7; and Henry, out of 196 examples, saw 4 in men; so that the proportion is as 1 to 42."

While this proportion is larger than my own cases indicate, the total number is so exceedingly small that cancer in the male breast must be classed among the extremely rare affections.

6 DDD

CHAPTER IX.

CANCER OF THE UTERUS—EARLY DIAGNOSIS
THE ONLY HOPE FOR THE PATIENT—THE
PRE-CANCEROUS STAGE—TREATMENT:
CAUSTICS; TOTAL EXTIRPATION—
DISINFECTANT FOR PA-
TIENT'S ROOM.

Twenty cases of cancer of the uterus, or less than
4 per cent. of the entire number, are recorded in my
table in Chapter XII. This is not to be regarded as
any index of the comparative frequency of the disease. Cancer of the uterus is usually discovered and
treated by the gynæcologist who is consulted for
what the patient supposes to be some ordinary uterine disease. In the New York Skin and Cancer Hospital, where there is a special clinic for internal cancer
in women, in 1890, twenty-two per cent. of all patients
with malignant disease were found to have cancer of
the uterus. In the Paris Register, among 8,289 fatal
cases of cancer, 2,996 were uterine, or upwards of
thirty-six per cent. This, however, may be taken
rather as a proof of the fatality of the disease in this
organ than of its relative frequency. On the other
hand, Satterthwaite's* percentage was four and eight-
tenths per cent.

---

* One Hundred Cases of Cancer.

One point is indisputable, after studying all the records before me, viz., that cancer of the uterus immediately follows malignant disease of the breast as to frequency, and outranks breast disease in its fatality. My number of cases (20) is not sufficient to render deductions of much scientific value, as several of them were absolutely incurable before they came under my care, but some general characteristics seem to be of sufficient importance to demand careful consideration.

In the first place, there is no class of cases where the disease is more likely to be undiscovered than in the uterus, and at the same time all hope of cure must be abandoned unless a diagnosis is made at the very earliest stage of the disease. Have we, with our present knowledge, any means of making this early diagnosis? Although Williams* has told us that it can be done by the aid of the microscope, especially when the suspected disease is in the portio vaginalis, still I doubt the possibility of making an accurate diagnosis in many cases, even by the most skillful pathologist. The anatomical division of the organ into the vaginal, cervical, and corporeal segments is of the greatest convenience for classification, but it is as useless as possible in determining how far the infiltration may have extended, for, from a clinical standpoint, the divisions are as imaginary as the imaginary lines upon

*Cancer of the Uterus: Harveian Lectures, 1886.

the page of a geographical atlas. As in the tongue we are never certain that cancer tissue has not been developed far beyond the apparently diseased portion, so in the uterus we have an organ with no natural barriers to even hinder the fatal progress of the malady. It is certainly true that clinical examination in these cases is less satisfactory than elsewhere, for the characteristic induration, such as belongs to cancer of the skin, for example, is often wanting until quite late in the history.

Subjective symptoms do not aid us oftentimes in making a diagnosis in the curable period of uterine cancer, if, indeed, there be such a period. A patient consulted me several years ago for a marked general debility, the cause of which I was for a time unable to discover. She complained of no pain, and gave no symptom pointing to disease of any special organ, until at last she incidentally remarked that sometimes she had a little leucorrhœa. An examination revealed the most extensive epithelioma of the vagina, portio vaginalis, and cervix which I have ever seen. From the osteum vaginæ in every direction, and almost filling the canal, was this enormous neoplasm of the most malignant type, which proved fatal a few weeks later. The patient had never suffered from pain, not even a backache. She was sixty-eight years of age, and I wish to repeat here what has been previously stated, that age is almost a determining factor in diagnosis. The ages of my twenty patients naturally divide them into two classes: 1. Those who were passing through the climacteric. 2. Women who had advanced some years beyond it. Their ages were as follows:

> Between 42 and 45................ .... 7 cases.
> Between 45 and 50................ ...... 6 cases.
> Between 50 and 60....... .... 6 cases.
> Between 60 and 70............... 1 case.

It will be observed that there was practically no case in the childbearing period, while between 42 and 50 years there were 13. The most important lesson to be learned from this fact is that a careful examination should always be made of a patient during this period, if her symptoms indicate, *in the slightest degree*, any ulcerating disease of the uterus. Any chronic inflammation of the cervix, or old laceration, or any cicatricial tissue, whether from pre-existing disease or as the result of operation, should be frequently and carefully examined. I include old lacerations in this list, notwithstanding Williams' statement that he has never seen cauliflower growth starting from a tear, and is of the opinion that laceration plays no part whatever in the ætiology of that form of cancer. There is no reason to doubt that a chronic irritation of the tissues here will prove an exciting cause of cancer during this period (between 40 and 50) just as surely as such a condition will cause an epithelioma of the lip, tongue, or skin.

In the case of patients between 50 and 70 years

of age, it may be said that a leucorrhœa or a metrorrhagia, however slight, is *usually* an indication of a
tendency to uterine cancer, if not of its actual exist-
ence. Sometimes a pessary will produce in old women
an ulceration of a pre-cancerous character. Such a
case has been under my care during the past two
years. The patient was 67 years old, and, although
the uterus had nearly disappeared, there was so much
relaxation of the vagina that she had worn a flexible
ring for a period of three years. It had not been removed in six months when she came to me with a
suspicious ulcer in Douglas' *cul de sac*, which, under
the most careful treatment with caustics, followed by
aristol dressings, was nearly a year in healing. This
leads me to repeat here what I have said elsewhere*
concerning aristol as an application in ulceration of
the uterus, both benign and malignant:

"A most satisfactory result of the use of aristol
powder was obtained in a number of cases of ulceration of the cervix uteri. It was applied by means of
an ordinary cotton tampon, smeared with vaseline, to
which the powder adhered, then placed in position
against the ulcer, and left from forty-eight to seventy-
two hours. Induration, thickening, and suppuration
were all promptly improved, and the ulcers, which
had resisted prolonged treatment by glycero-tannin,
borated solutions, and other applications in common
use, finally healed. In no case was any irritation excited by the remedy itself, the stimulating effect cor-

responding in degree to that of tincture of iron used in similar cases.

"Another application in these cases, which is convenient and efficacious, is a mixture of aristol and iodol in equal parts, applied through the speculum by an ordinary powder blower, after which a light tampon of absorbent cotten may be inserted."

The treatment of cancer of the uterus, when of a pronounced character, is usually of no permanent benefit. We should, however, attempt to cure the patient, especially if the disease seems to be confined to the portio vaginalis. I have attempted it in such cases by removal of the cervix and cauterizing with ter-chloride of antimony, the Paquelin cautery, and other agents, sometimes preceding their use by thorough curetting far beyond the internal os, and yet in none of my cases was an immunity from disease secured lasting over six months. In one case the entire uterus was removed by a skillful operator two months before the patient entered my service, and even in that short period a recurrent growth, the size of a fœtal head, filled the entire pelvic cavity. It appeared to have originated in the parametrium, in the neighborhood of both broad ligaments. I am obliged to confess that all my twenty patients are dead, with one exception, and she has only been under observation the last few weeks, and is going to follow the others in a few

* New York Medical Record, June 6th, 1892.

months. As sad as my histories are, all my colleagues, as far as my personal knowledge extends, have an equally dismal report to make of the final results in their cases.

We should not close this chapter, however, without referring to some of the brilliant immediate results of ablation of the uterus for cancer. In the first place, removal of the uterus should never be attempted if the disease has extended beyond the uterus itself. Under any circumstances, especially for the determination of that point, *an examination should be made under an anæsthetic.*

The fatality of the operation of total extirpation has been somewhat lessened as surgeons have become more familiar with it, but it is still enormous. Freund, of Strassburg, lost seventy-two per cent. as a result of the operation, but Schrœder has reported forty cases with a mortality of only ten. Now, note the subsequent history of his remaining cases:

14 had a respite of.................	I year.
8 " " "	1½ years.
4 " " "	2 "
2 " " "	3 "
1 " " "	3½ "
1 " " "	4 ',
30	

The last one died of apoplexy without recurrence of cancer. Here we find an average interval between the operation and recurrence (and they all had recurrence, except the one who escaped through an apoplexy) of between two and three years. Several of them might have lived that length of time without any treatment. We had a case in the Skin and Cancer Hospital which lasted over four years without any treatment beyond disinfecting douches, and the last months of her life were peaceful and painless.

For the purpose of disinfecting the room occupied by cancer patients, in several instances I have used with satisfaction the following plan, suggested by Dr. H. Gesould, of Cleveland, Ohio: Dissolve 12. grammes of nitrate of potash in 250. grammes of Platt's chlorides, full strength. In this saturate thin muslin, and burn it in the room and under the bed-clothing as often as required. Its use causes no discomfort to the attendants or offensive odor in adjoining rooms.

CHAPTER X.

CANCER OF THE RECTUM—HISTORY OF A CASE—VARIETIES OF—CAUSATION—EXAMINATION OF RECTUM—SYMPTOMS—TREATMENT—CARE OF INCURABLE CASES.

Cancer of the rectum is not of frequent occurrence, only one per cent. of my own cases being in that location. In Marsden's table of 10,759 cases of cancer treated in the London Cancer Hospital,* 61 were in the rectum, being slightly above one-half of one per cent. This table agrees with all others in showing a very large preponderance of males, the proportion being about six to one.

The history of the following case illustrates the points which we wish to discuss in this chapter:

Mr. A. H., sixty years of age, a farmer by occupation, has always been healthy until eighteen months ago. He never had piles, or fistula, or fissure, all of which are often predisposing causes of cancer. Neither does he give any family history of malignant disease or phthisis. His facial expression is that of a man suffering with severe constitutional disease. His appetite and digestion are poor, and he tells me he

---

*Marsden on Cancer.

has lost forty pounds in weight since the trouble began.

His first symptom was an obstinate diarrhœa, which resisted all the usual treatment, and continues at present, it being usual for him to have a passage as often as every hour during the day. There is little pain during the stools, and only slight traces of blood have occasionally been noticed.

The pain, which is now almost constant, he describes as a burning and heavy pain across the loins, extending down the back of the thighs, and he complains of difficult, painful micturition, due, of course, to the disease of the prostate and bladder. Physical examination reveals nothing wrong until the finger is passed high up into the rectum, when we find in front the enlarged and tender prostate, and behind it a projecting growth, greatly resembling a cervix uteri, with a small opening in the center, into which the finger can be passed with difficulty—all there is left of the rectal canal. Behind this is a cul-de-sac, which makes the similarity to the cervix complete.

It is impossible to say how high the disease extends, but it is evident that the beginning is more than four inches from the anus. The importance of this fact will appear when we consider the treatment. There are no diseased glands in the groin or elsewhere.

VARIETIES.

Cancer of the rectum may be either carcinoma, usually scirrhous (or, as Purcell calls it, scirrhoid*), or epithelioma. Allingham† mentions two cases of so-called rodent ulcer of the rectum, one a carcinoma and the other an epithelial growth.

I find no authentic records of a *primary* sarcoma of the rectum. One case of secondary sarcoma in my own practice was interesting. The patient, a woman of 42 years, had a sarcoma of the rectum, which began in the connective tissue between the sacrum and the rectum. That, in itself, was not very remarkable, for Mr. Purcell, in speaking of sarcomas contiguous to bone, says that "the places of selection in which these tumors appear are about the lower end of the femur and upper end of the tibia, and they are not uncommon at the upper part of the thigh, and about the pelvis." This tumor was discovered early, attention having been called thereto by the pain. When first examined it was attached to the periosteum, was about the size of a hen's egg, and had pushed the rectum to one side somewhat. It increased rapidly, pain became constant, and the rectum was soon infiltrated with the disease. About this time the patient became pregnant, and, to our dismay, did not miscarry. She refused to have an induced labor, and at term it was

---

* Purcell, Cancer and Its Treatment
† Allingham, Diseases of the Rectum.

a question whether delivery could be accomplished. Prof. Thomas was called in consultation, and finally decided to try delivery by version. After turning, very firm compression was made upon the abdomen in the direction of the uterine axis, and a nearly asphyxiated, small-sized child was delivered, which is now twelve years of age. After her recovery, Dr. Erskine Mason, who was a judicious advocate of lumbar colotomy in such cases, was called in, but did not advise the operation as long as fæces could be evacuated by enemata, and she died of exhaustion one and a half years from the beginning of the disease, without operation.

CAUSATION.

Cook* mentions cancer of the rectum as being developed after some operations for piles, which is of an unusually malignant character. It is doubtless true that piles should be mentioned among the predisposing causes of rectal cancer, as well as fistula, fissure of the anus, and syphilitic disease. As we have often noted in diseases of other organs, so here, any prolonged irritation of mucous membrane is liable to induce cancerous degeneration of epithelium.

EXAMINATION.

The examination of a patient for rectal cancer should be conducted with especial reference to the comfort of the patient as far as that can be done

* T. W. Cook, Cancer; Its Allies and Counterfeits.

without inaccuracy of diagnosis. "Sims' position" is the only one which is really satisfactory to both doctor and patient. If any rectal speculum is to be employed it should be the one devised by Sims for rectal use, but experience has confirmed my opinion that only one instrument should ever be employed for this purpose, and that is the index finger. A trained sense of touch fixes the location, extent, variety and complications of cancer of the rectum so thoroughly that the sense of sight is of no value afterwards. It can be far more easily introduced than a speculum, causes less pain, and is free from the danger of rupturing the diseased tissue and thereby doing unlimited damage.

SYMPTOMS.

A careful study of the case heretofore narrated furnishes several of the prominent symptoms of rectal cancer, but Walsh* gives such a graphic description of them that I will quote his exact words:

"The symptoms differ in the early stage, according to the form under which the affection occurs. The greater the amount of pressure on nerves, the more severe will be the pain. A sensation of uneasiness in the rectum, a feeling as if its contents were never thoroughly evacuated, and a consequent repetition of the act of defecation, twice or more in the same day, sometimes accompanied with tenesmus, are

---

* Nature and Treatment of Cancer.

among the first effects of the disease. These incon-
veniences may have possibly existed for a considerable
time before the morbid deposition has proceeded to
any extent; the nature of the disease is at that time
rarely suspected; difficulty in defecation progressively
increases; a discharge of pus, or muco-pus, frequently
accompanies that of the fæces, which are more or less
tinged with blood; the latter may be effused in large
quantities, but this is not common. Obstinate constipation, alternating with profuse diarrhœa, the
former lasting four days, while the accumulation of
flatus and fæces swells the abdomen to an enormous
size, now becomes a formidable symptom. The copious evacuation eventually brought about either by
purgatives or by the natural irritation of acrid secretions, leaves the patient in a state of extreme collapse,
and a prolonged fainting fit is not uncommon under
the circumstances. Before this relief occurs the
symptoms may have become those of internal strangulation—nausea, vomiting of fæciform matter, hic-
cough, coldness of the extremities, vertigo, and even
delirium. Irritation is meanwhile set up in the neigh-
boring parts, and difficult micturition, or in some
cases, on the contrary, incontinence of urine, follows.
Irritability of the bladder may, indeed (but this is
rare), be the earliest annoyance experienced by the
patient.

"Abscesses sometimes form around the intestine,
and burst into the vagina in females—an occurrence

which sometimes produces much relief from the facility which it affords for the passage of the fæces. In males such abscesses open into the bladder or urethra, in which case the patient voids both flatus and feculent matter by that route. In advanced cases there is œdema of the genitals and lower extremities. Unless relieved by the formation of an artificial opening in the bowel, the symptoms increase in violence; the retention of the intestinal contents becomes complete; not even flatus escapes; extreme tympanitis ensues, with the symptoms of a strangulation; a rupture of the bowel from fæcal and flatulent distension occurs, followed by fatal effusion into the peritoneum."

Walsh says nothing about the peculiar odor of the discharges from cancer of the rectum, which some authors believe to be pathognomonic.

TREATMENT.

The treatment of cancer of the rectum may be either curative or palliative. The only cases in which caustic treatment is even admissible are those rare instances where a protruding mass at the anus and extending a very short distance into the rectum may be removed by caustic potash or the actual cautery.

When the disease does not extend more than four or five inches from the anus, with no infected glands in the lumbar or vaginal region, extirpation by operation may cure your patient. In other words, the same rule which I have given you in regard to operations in other localities applies here, viz.: *An operation for cancer is only justifiable when there is a fair prospect that every vestige of diseased tissue can be removed.*

Palliative measures are called for to relieve the constipation, the pain, and the extremely disagreeable odor of the discharges.

Laxatives will be required very often, and should be such as will act without causing irritation. The compound liquorice powder is quite satisfactory oftentimes.

One compound rhubarb pill every four hours has recently given one of my patients great relief, after nearly all other laxatives had been exhausted.

In giving enemas let me suggest the attaching of the largest size soft rubber catheter to the nozzle of the syringe, which can then be passed far into the rectum without the slightest pain or inconvenience to the patient. Do not distend the bowels with fluid in an advanced case, for fear of rupture.

When all else fails, lumbar colotomy is our only remedy. It is a desperate remedy, often proves fatal, and when successful, the period of relief is brief. I always question whether our duty as surgeons requires us to undertake, or even justifies us in performing, an operation, which at best can only prolong a life whose possessor usually prays for a final rest.

Dilatation by the finger or a soft rubber bougie

7 DDD

by a very careful hand has sometimes proved very useful in my cases. None but the surgeon himself or a careful nurse should undertake the operation. *Never* allow the patient himself to pass an instrument into the rectum.

Your experience with opiates will suggest numerous forms and methods to employ for relieving pain. Continue your efforts to relieve this symptom until you succeed, if possible. The patient will thoroughly appreciate your efforts.

The diet should be highly concentrated, and not highly seasoned. Murdock's liquid food is among the best of the recently offered preparations.

For allaying fœtor, frequent bathing and an occasional injection of a solution of sulphate of copper (4. to 250.) are useful. Then let the patient wear a pad of soft oakum, held in place by a T-bandage. A thin layer of softer material may be placed next to the skin.

All that has been attempted here is to indicate the lines which the management of these cases should follow.

The operations of extirpation and colotomy are nowhere better described than in Cripp's and Allingham's excellent books on "Diseases of the Rectum."

CHAPTER XI.

UNUSUAL CASES OF CANCER—SARCOMA OF SCALP—EPITHELIOMA INVOLVING WRIST JOINT—EPITHELIOMA OF BACK OF HAND—EXCISION OF THE BREAST UNDER COCAINE.

SARCOMA OF SCALP.

The patient with sarcoma of the scalp, which is represented in the cut (*vide* frontispiece), was a girl fourteen years of age. In infancy she was severely burned on the head, and when she was seven years old received a cut upon the same place. About two years after, a tumor developed in the cicatrix. This was removed by caustic, and four times was removed by operation during the following six years Then she was referred to me, and in the meantime the ulceration had destroyed the entire skin over an area of nearly thirty square inches, while in the central and deepest portion the bone had been destroyed, so that the intra-cranial pulsation was distinctly seen and readily counted. The borders of this enormous ulcer were elevated, everted, and hard, the disease spreading in all directions. Notwithstanding all this disease existing six years, the girl was well nourished, extremely intelligent, and apparently in excellent health. The most conspicuous symptom was extreme pain whenever the surface was exposed to the air, either warm or cold. Alveloz was applied several times to the surface, but with no benefit. Further operation was out of the question. The most comfortable dressing was the following, which serves well for many extensive malignant ulcers:

> ℞ Cretæ preparatæ........... 12.
> Ol. amygdalæ dulcis........ 8.
> Misc. et add.
> Lanolin .... 60.
> Sig. Apply twice daily, spread upon lint.

The patient died of what was called malarial fever a few months after leaving the hospital.

A man, forty years of age, was admitted to my service in the New York Skin and Cancer Hospital, Dec. 19th, 1887, with an enormous cancerous ulcer of the scalp, covering the same portion as in the case just mentioned, which began as a tumor of the skin behind the left ear, ten years before. Sections from several portions of the elevated border of the ulcer showed the growth to be a sarcoma. Before admission, it had been often treated both by operation and by various caustic applications. A striking peculiarity marked its invasion of new tissue: First, the skin became blue and swollen in a manner resembling varicose veins, although of firm texture. This was followed by a change to a firm lardy patch, so nearly like morphœa that some who saw the patient before the microscopical examination had been made believed it to be an anomalous case of that disease. Thus the disease gradually extended, chiefly in the direction of the forehead and occiput. The head was finally drawn firmly toward the left shoulder, the left ear became œdematous, the pain in and around the ulcer increased, a sarcoma appeared in the scrotum, and when the patient died of exhaustion, two years later, some cancer was found in the spleen and liver. He was a miner by occupation, of strong build, had never had syphilis, and gave no history of any injury, neither was there any family history of cancer. Both these cases were so remarkable that I give them a place here on account of their rarity, for they were of course not suitable cases for active treatment.

EPITHELIOMA INVOLVING THE WRIST JOINT.

A patient, fifty-five years of age, was referred to me by my colleague, Dr. George H. Fox, who, six years before, had a small epithelioma upon the back of the left wrist, directly over the joint. It finally ulcerated, and upon admission the disease was about five square inches in extent, of irregular shape, indurated edges, and the central portion had invaded the joint, where diseased bone was easily discovered. Amputation of the forearm near the elbow was performed, and resulted in a cure. Two years afterwards there had been no recurrence.

EPITHELIOMA OF THE BACK OF THE HAND.

An Englishman, sixty years of age, applied for admission to the hospital, upon the back of whose right hand was a large, cauliflower-like· tumor (sarcoma), which sprang from a base about one inch in diameter. In the central portion it was three-quarters of an inch high, and sloped gradually to the borders, which were quite thin, and rested upon the back of the hand throughout the entire circumference of the growth. The entire surface was raw, and bled considerably, even when handled carefully. The first appearance of the disease was six years before, and it had been several times removed in a London hospital. I first removed it with Bougard's paste. The slough separated, leaving an apparently healthy base, but in six weeks new cancerous disease had developed in the cicatrix. It was then removed by operation— as we believed, thoroughly. A few weeks later he returned to London, and I referred him to Mr. Henry Morris, of the Middlesex Hospital, who afterwards informed me that the disease was developing in the forearm, and the arm was to be amputated. The extreme malignancy of this tumor was remarkable. I am not able to give the final termination of the case, but have no doubt it has ended disastrously.

During the past autumn (1891) a woman, seventy-five years old, was admitted to my service, with a tumor so nearly resembling the one just related that the same description may be applied to it, except regarding the degree of malignancy. It had been of slow growth, had existed six years, but had never been treated. It caused very slight pain, and the same was true of the former case. This was removed by Bougard's paste, healed kindly, and three months afterwards there had been no recurrence.

AMPUTATION OF THE BREAST UNDER COCAINE.

In 1886 I exhibited the following case before the Surgical Section of the New York Academy of Medicine. The patient was a woman, seventy-eight years of age, and a native of Scotland. A tumor of the right breast was discovered by her six years previously. It had increased slowly but steadily in size until the entire breast was involved, and for several months ulceration had existed in the most prominent part of the growth. There were no enlarged axillary glands. The patient was in fair health, with the important exception of having an enlarged heart, with both aortic and mitral insufficiency. The prognosis regarding an operation was good, but ether was strongly contra-indicated. It was, therefore, determined to employ cocaine. The field of operation was surrounded by one of the rubber rings devised by Dr. J. Leonard Corning for preventing the rapid dissemination of cocaine, and the lines of incision were very thoroughly injected with a two-per-cent. solution. By the aid of a long needle the base of the tumor was also anæsthetized. Twenty minutes were required for the operation. She talked of her old Scotch home during the entire time, and never felt the slightest pain until the very last horse-hair suture was being introduced. Primary union resulted, and three years later there had been no recurrence. Several months afterwards a removal of the breast under cocaine was reported in the London Lancet, the operator claiming it to be the first and only time the operation had been thus attempted. That such an operation may be successfully performed is thus proved, and in case the heart is diseased, and the patient far advanced in years, it may be of the greatest value. Dr. Corning's ingenious invention was of the greatest value here, as I have found it to be in many other cases in which his plan has been adopted.

CHAPTER XII.

REMARKS ON THE AUTHOR'S CASES—LOCATION OF THE DISEASE—ASSIGNED CAUSES— RESULTS—IS CANCER A FEBRILE DISEASE?—BIBLIOGRAPHY.

The consideration of the following tables of my 534 cases, in which an accurate record has been made, will be interesting to the investigator of the natural history of cancer in three particulars, viz., in reference to the sex and age of patients, the assigned influence of heredity (by the patient), and the various traumatic influences, which have been carefully investigated and only mentioned where I have satisfied myself that the injury was a probable ætiological factor in the case. Whenever the patient has reported that any relative, near or remote, has suffered from cancer, heredity has been mentioned as an assigned cause, but it is proper to state that in a vast majority of cases the probable influence of heredity is extremely doubtful. Of the entire number only *two* gave a marked and indisputable history of a hereditary tendency. It should be noted that the tables are arranged in the order of frequency of development in the different organs or regions affected, and, as usual, breast cases head the list.

DISEASES LOCATED IN THE BREAST.

Total number.. 141
Females... 140
Males.......   1
Maximum age... 75
Minimum age... 20
Average age... 48½
Right breast.. 78
Left breast... 63

Assigned Causes.

Heredity 15 cases.......................... 10 per cent.
Blow 24 cases.............................. 17   "   "
Paget's disease 2 cases................... 1⅖   "   "
Wart 2 cases.............................. 1⅖   "   "

The one patient, aged 20, suffered from a cystic sarcoma of the right breast, which had been treated as a mammary abscess. A blow was the cause. A maternal aunt had cancer of the breast. Operation on November 4, 1888, and three and a half years afterwards there has been no recurrence.

Two of the number had recurrent disease in the remaining breast, one three months after operation, and the other three and a half years after removal. In the first instance the recurrent disease was promptly removed, but the patient developed a multitude of cancerous tumors in and around both cicatrices, and death occurred in five months after the primary operation.

FACE.

Total number	70
Females	29
Males..	41
Maximum age	87
Minimum age	8
Average age	57

Assigned Causes.

Heredity, 2 cases............................	3 per cent.
Blow, 3 cases	4	"
Cut, 5 cases.................................	7	"

In the above table, epithelioma affecting special organs—eyelids, nose, and lips—are not included. Whenever the disease was of small area, not exceeding four square inches, it was treated by a caustic plaster, either Marsden's or Bougard's paste. Recurrence has been exceedingly rare, and we are amply justified in the opinion that 90 per cent. are permanently cured. I have no doubt that every case could be cured if the treatment were commenced at the very beginning of the disease. One of the most satisfactory results of the treatment by these caustics is the absence of any noticeable cicatrix.

LOWER LIP.

Total number	62
Females	7
Males..	55
Maximum age.................................	82
Minimum age	26
Average age..................................	55

Assigned Causes.

Heredity, 5 cases.............................. 8 per cent.
Smoking, 13 cases............................ 21   "
Tooth, 3 cases 5   "
Burn, 2 cases 3   "
Cut, 1 case.
Glass-blowing, 1 case.

The glass-blower had recurrent disease twice after an apparent cure, but finally changed his occupation, and after eight years remains well. The small number of female patients should be noted.

NOSE.

Total number 43
Females 19
Males... 24
Maximum age.. 78
Minimum age.. 32
Average age 60

Assigned Causes.

Heredity, 3 cases........................... 7   per cent.
Blow, 2 cases .... 4½   "
Wart, 5 cases .... 11½   "
Glasses, 1 case........................... 2   "

The patient who assigned the disease to his eye-glasses wore the ordinary eye-glass for several years, and an indurated point developed just where the pressure of the bow compressed the skin on the left side of the nose. The cork protective now placed upon such glasses will probably prevent such an accident.

TONGUE.

Total number.. 34
Females... 3
Males... 31
Maximum age.. 64
Minimum age.. 30
Average age.. 52

Assigned Causes.

Heredity, 3 cases.............................. 9 per cent.
Smoking, 7 cases.............................. 20 per cent.
Sharp tooth, 10 cases .... 29 per cent.

The fact that a larger percentage was attributed to the irritation of a tooth than to smoking, it will be noticed, is decided, as well as the extremely small proportion of females who developed cancer in this organ.

EYELID AND ORBIT.

Total number... 23
Females.. 11
Males.. 12
Maximum age... 81
Minimum age.. 9
Average age.. 54

Assigned Causes.

Heredity, 1 case.............................. 4 per cent.
Wart, 3 cases................................. 13 per cent.
Blow, 1 case.................................. 4 per cent.

UTERUS.

Total number... 23
Maximum age.. 70
Minimum age.. 35
Average age.. 50

Assigned Causes.

Heredity, 2 cases............................ 9 per cent.
Injury, 1 case............................... 4 per cent.

Only one of these patients was unmarried, and all the others had been delivered of one or more children. The injury above mentioned was a severe fall, and a supra-pubic blow caused soreness which never disappeared, the disease developing in the body of the uterus.

NECK.

Total number.. 22
Females... 5
Males... 17
Maximum age.. 70
Minimum age.. 22
Average age.. 46

Assigned Causes.

Wart, 1 case............................... 4½ per cent.
Cut, 1 case............................... 4½ "

JAW.

Total number.. 16
Females... 6
Males 10
Maximum age.. 68
Minimum age.. 18
Average age 43
Upper jaw 2
Lower jaw 14

Assigned Causes.

Heredity, 1 case............................ 6 per cent.
Smoking, 1 case............................ 6 "
Sharp tooth, 1 case .... 6 "

The patient aged 18 was a woman who had what was thought to be a non-malignant epulis for several years, which finally developed malignancy, and proved to be a sarcoma. There has been no recurrence six years after operating.

FOREHEAD.

Total number	13
Females	9
Males	4
Maximum age	74
Minimum age	28
Average age	53

Assigned Causes.

Wart, 1 case	7 per cent.

All these cases were treated by caustic plaster, and the cure was permanent in every instance.

RECTUM.

Total number	12
Females	3
Males	9
Maximum age	75
Minimum age	44
Average age	55

Assigned Causes.

Heredity, 1 case	8 per cent.
Contusion, 1 case	8 "

HEAD.

Total number	9
Females	3
Males	6
Maximum age	74
Minimum age	14
Average age	59

Assigned Causes.

Blow, 1 case................................... 11 per cent.
Burn, 1 case 11   "

Two of these patients had wens, in one of which
the cancer developed after an injury of the cyst,
which caused severe inflammation; the other developed the disease at the base of the wen, without any
known exciting cause.

MOUTH.

Total number.................................... 7
Females.. 4
Males.. 3
Maximum age.................................... 67
Minimum age.................................... 18
Average age..................................... 43

Assigned Causes.

Sharp tooth, 3 cases.......................... 42 per cent.
Smoking, 1 case............................... 14   "   "

HAND.

Total number.................................... 6
Females.. 1
Males.. 5
Maximum age.................................... 75
Minimum age.................................... 40
Average age..................................... 59

No causes were assigned in these cases. The
disease appeared on the back of the hand in most of
them. One proved to be an exceedingly malignant
sarcoma, which has been fully described in Chapter
XI.

STOMACH.

Total number........ 5
Females.. 4
Males... I
Maximum age...................................... 58
Minimum age... 35
Average age....................................... 48

This record gives us only $\frac{9}{10}$ per cent. of cancer of the stomach. There is a wide difference of opinion regarding the frequency of cancer of the stomach. I am inclined to the belief that in New York, at least, it is extremely infrequent. At the Demilt Dispensary, where I had charge of the class for diseases of the digestive organs, in five years only one case of cancer of the stomach applied for treatment, although over 10,000 patients were treated during that period. Mr. Jessett declares that "this organ yields to the uterus alone in the frequency with which it is attacked by cancer." He arrives at this conclusion from a study of various statistics, which are not trustworthy indices of the actual number, for an autopsy is often necessary to make a diagnosis of cancer of the stomach. One of my cases of cancer of the œsophagus was referred to me as cancer of the stomach, the post-mortem examination of which proved the stomach to be perfectly free from disease. I would not dare to make a positive diagnosis of cancer of the stomach unless careful palpation revealed the presence of a tumor.

8 DDD

ŒSOPHAGUS.

Total number..... 4
Females 1
Males... 3
Maximum age....................................... 72
Minimum age....................................... 48
Average age....................................... 50

EXTERNAL EAR.

Total number...................... 3
Females... 1
Males... 2
Maximum age....................................... 83
Minimum age....................................... 50
Average age....................................... 92

Assigned Causes.

Frost-bite, 1 case......................... 33 per cent.
Scratch with comb, 1 case................. 33   "

Of cancer of the larynx I had 1 case, age 49; of the liver, 2 cases, ages 72 and 60; of the omentum, 2 cases, ages 53 and 31; of the foot, 1 case, age 63; and miscellaneous, 30 cases, ages 76 to 14.

RECAPITULATION.

Total number..................................... 534
Females... 287
Males... 247
Maximum age....................................... 81
Minimum age....................................... 8
History of heredity............................... 33
History of injury................................. 64

IS CANCER A FEBRILE DISEASE?

There are several features of the natural history of cancer which suggest the possibility of its being a febrile disease. The similarities to the process of simple inflammation in many cases and the gradual but continuous emaciation, in many instances, even when the disease is still local, indicate the possible truth of this hypothesis. Raymond and Brodeur reported a case in La France Médicale, in 1883, in a man aged 76, in which no primary cancer could be discovered. There were disseminated hard nodules, from the size of a pea to a bean, which the microscope showed to be genuine carcinoma. The growths from the pericardium, pleura, and peritoneum had essentially the same structure. There was a tumor in the liver which was declared to be a cavernous angeioma. The symptoms during life were similar to those of pulmonary tuberculosis. *There were periodical febrile attacks, simulating ague.*

In 1887, W. Ebstein published (in the Berlin. klin. Wochenschrift, No. 31) a case which was characterized by alternating periods of high fever and apyrexia, and when, exhausted by increasing weakness, the patient finally died, the disease proved to be malignant lympho-sarcoma.

The editor of the Lancet for January 16, 1892, after referring to Ebstein's case, gives the following history, published by C. Paritz, of a case observed in the clinic of Dr. Tschudnowsky at St. Petersburg:

"The patient was a young man, twenty-two years of age, who, in the autumn of 1889, began to suffer from increasing weakness, dyspnœa, and enlargement of the abdomen. Examination showed the presence of some nodular masses in the abdomen, contiguous to the liver, but it could not be determined whether they were actually connected with that organ; also some enlargement of the spleen and of the axillary and cervical glands. There was also marked anæmia. Four years previously he had acquired a sore on the penis, but this had not been followed by any syphilitic signs, and it may at once be said that the supposition that the conditions were due to syphilitic infection was negatived by the failure of anti-syphilitic treatment to modify the course of his illness. In February, 1890, he began to be febrile, and during the next six months he had several attacks of fever, uninfluenced by quinine, with intervals of freedom from pyrexia. It was in August that he came to the St. Petersburg clinic, and the case was carefully observed to its close in November. It was throughout marked by a high degree of fever, of an irregularly remittent and intermittent type, wholly uncontrolled by antiseptic remedies, arsenic, or other drugs. The masses in the abdomen were thought to be connected with mesenteric and retro-peritoneal glands, and the diagnosis of lympho-sarcoma was made. The anæmia and weakness increased, and death was preceded by peritonitis. At the post-mortem examination the liver was found to be enormously enlarged and the seat of numerous soft whitish masses of new growth, some of which had broken down, whilst the lymphatic glands in the abdomen were unaffected. The spleen was enlarged, as also were the cervical and axillary glands, which had been noticed during life."

As a slight contribution to this hitherto unexplored field, we have systematically recorded the temperature in a series of inoperative cases of cancer. In none of them was there a suppurative process to account for variations in temperature. The most notable example is that of a patient who was admitted to the hospital March 3, 1888, suffering from dermatitis herpetiformis. He also had alopecia areata, but these diseases were slight, and could in no degree account for the steadily downward course of the patient, who died May 1.1. The autopsy revealed very extensive sarcomatous deposits in the abdominal organs—liver, spleen, mesenteric glands, etc. His temperature chart from the date of admission was as follows, taken under the tongue:

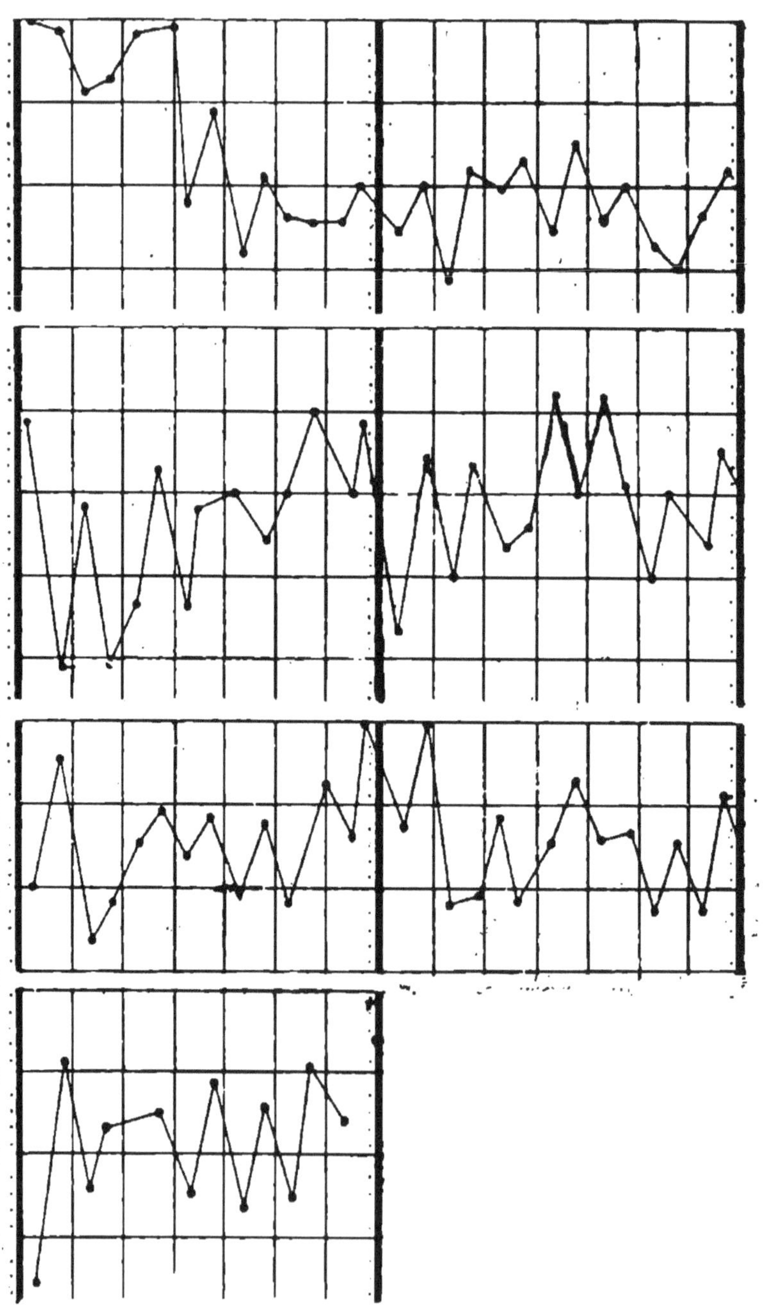
100
99
98
97
100
99
98
97
100
99
98
99
98
97

The following record is from a case of epithelioma of the tongue which was never operated upon, owing to the infection of the sub-lingual glands. These indicate axillary, instead of sublingual, temperature, and cover the time from his admission, Jan. 10, 1889, until his death, which occurred March 2, of the same year.

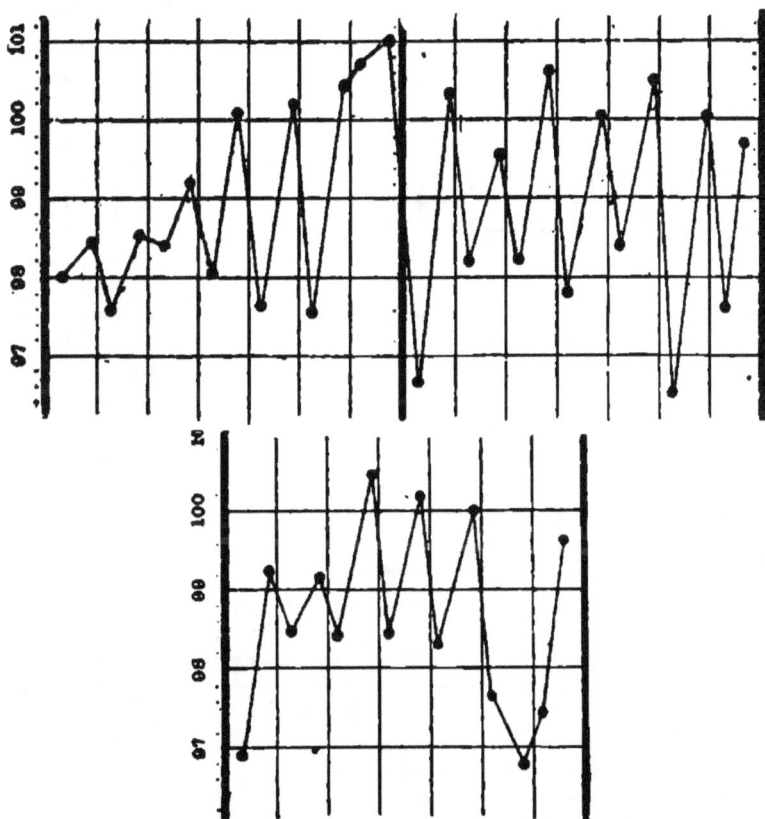

The next record of axillary temperature is from a patient, aged 63, with cancer of the uterus and vagina, showing a decided and pretty regular curve, but the actual temperature remaining low.

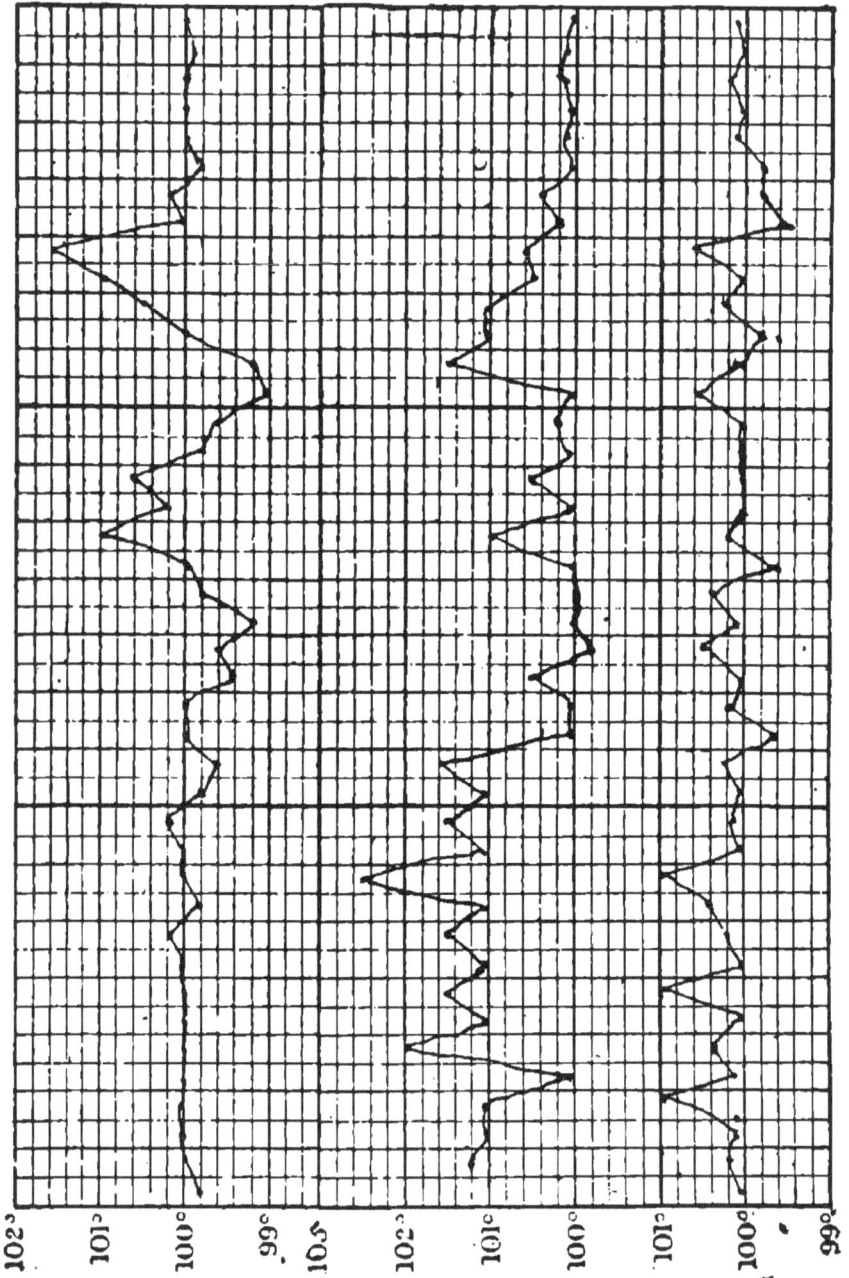

Mrs. Q., aged 36, with a general carcinosis for three weeks preceding death from exhaustion, furnished the following:

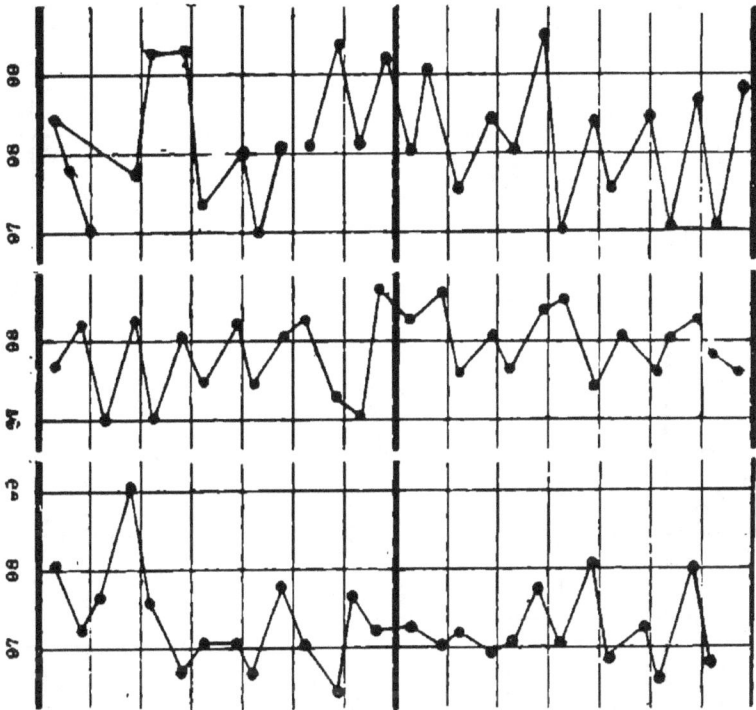

A man, aged 41, whose case has been referred to, with a immense sarcomatous ulcer of the scalp, and in whom the disease was found to be considerably disseminated at death, had marked and constant fluctuations in temperature for ten weeks preceding death, which was due to exhaustion. His chart is as follows:

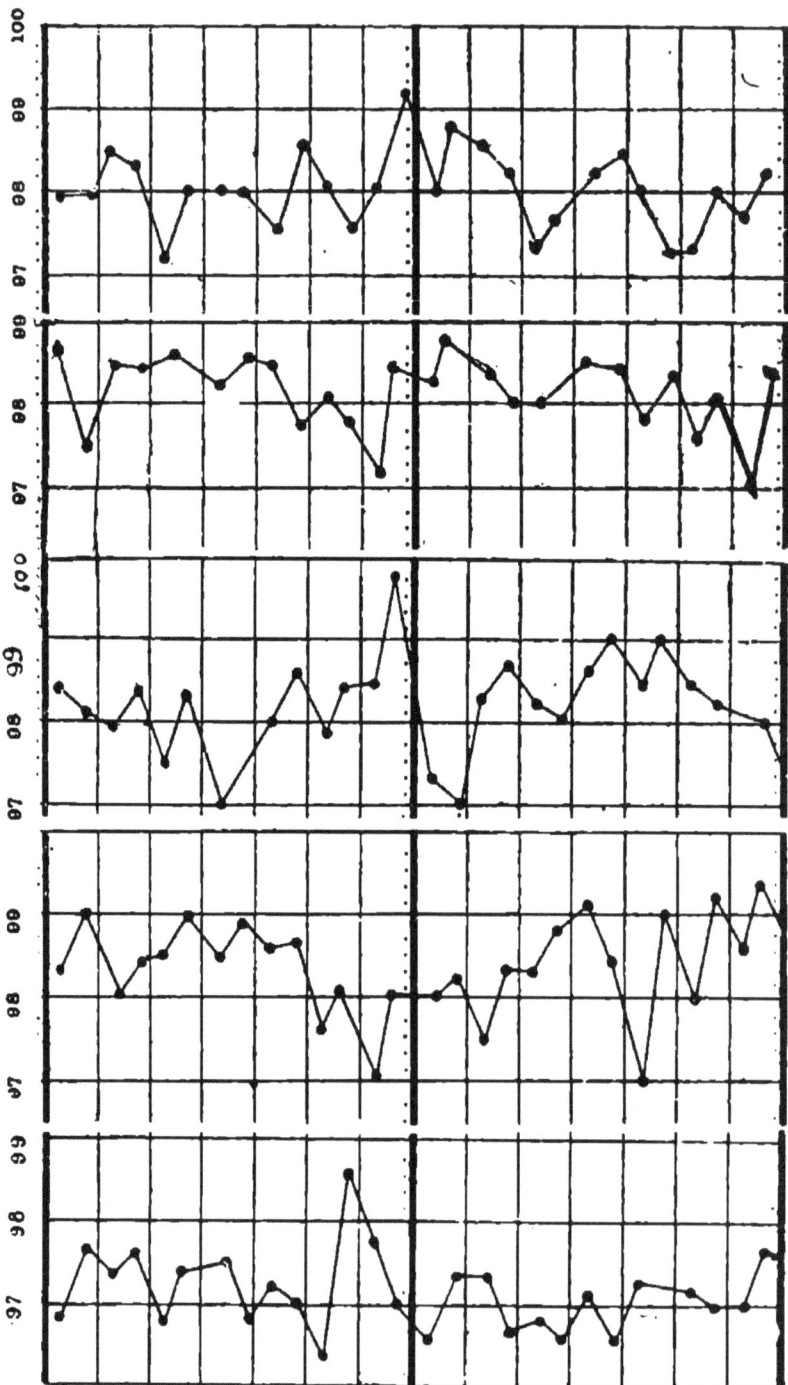

Other records indicate, as do those above given, a decided febrile movement, when there is a general dissemination of the disease. There seems to be no evidence of such a condition while the disease remains a strictly local one. The question remains, like so many others connected with the study of diseases, a field for the investigator, which may yield results of decided value.

BIBLIOGRAPHY.

Adams, Joseph: Cancerous Breast, London, 1801; Observations on Morbid Poisons; Phagedæna and Cancer, London, 1795.

Agnew, C. R., and David Webster: Sarcoma—Enucleations of Eyeball, Reprint from Ophthalmic Journal, July 1891.

Aldis, Sir Charles: Glandular Diseases, Especially Cancer, London, 1832.

Allingham, William: Diseases of Rectum, London, 1882.

Althouse, J.: Electrolytic Treatment of Tumors, London, 1867.

Arnott, Henry: Cancer—Varieties, Histology, and Diagnosis, London, 1871.

Ball, Charles B.: Diseases and Treatment of the Rectum and Anus, London, 1887.

Bell, Benjamin: Treatment on the Hydrocele, on Sarcocele, or Cancer of the Testes, Edinburgh, 1794.

Bennett, James Risdon: Cancer and other Intra-Thoracic Growths, London, 1872.

Bennett, J. Hughes: Cancerous and Cancroid Growths, Edinburgh, 1849.

Birchmore, W. N.: Cancer in Lower Animals (Manuscript).

Birket, John: Diseases of the Breast, London, 1850.

Broca, Paul: Traité des Tumeurs, Paris, 1866.

Bryant, Thomas: Diseases of the Breast, London, 1887.

Butlin, Henry T.: Operative Surgery of Malignant Diseases, London, 1887; Sarcoma and Carcinoma, London, 1882; Diseases of the Tongue, Philadelphia, 1885; Diseases of the Rectum and Anus, London, 1884; Malignant Disease of Larynx, London, 1884.

Carmichael, Richard: Effects of Carbonate and Other Preparations of Iron upon Cancer, Dublin, 1809.

Churchill, John Francis: Increase of Cancer in England, and Cause, London, 1885. This contains some valuable statistics.

Clay, John: Treatment of Cancer by Chian Turpentine, London, 1882.

Collis, Maurice Henry: Cancer and Tumors, London, 1864.

Conquoin, A.: Traitement du Cancer, Paris, 1838.

Cooke, Thos. Weeden: Cancer, its Allies and Counterfeits, London, 1865.

Creighton, Chas.: Physiology and Pathology of the Breast, London, 1878.

Cripps, W. Harrison: Cancer of the Rectum, London, 1880; Passage of Air and Fæces from the Urethra, London, 1888.

Currier, A. F.: Cancer of the Uterus, Reprint from New York Medical Journal, March 5, 1887.

Delevan, D. Bryson: Primary Epithelioma of the Tonsil, Reprint from New York Medical Journal, April, 1882.

De Morgan, Campbell: On Cancer, London, 1872; Use of Chloride of Zinc in Operations for Removal of Cancerous Tumors, London, 1866.

Edgelow: New Electrolytic Treatment of Cancer, London, 1879.

Fell, J. Weldon: Treatise on Cancer, London, 1857; Treatment of Cancer by Means of Paste and Incisions, London, 1866.

Fox, W. T. & T. C.: Rodent Ulcer, London, 1879 (Pamphlet).

Gross, Samuel W.: Practical Treatise on Tumors of the Mammary Gland, New York, 1880.

Haldane, D. Rutherford Co-existence of Tubercle and Cancer, Edinburgh, 1872.

Hickman, W.: Cancerous Diseases of Bone, London, 1865.

Home, Sir Everard, Bart.; Short Tract on Formation of Tumors, London, 1830; Observations on Cancer, London, 1805.

Howard, John: Practical Observations on Cancer, London, 1811.

Jennings, Charles Egerton: Excision of Cancer of Entire Uterus, London, 1886; Cancer and its Complications, London, 1889.

Jessett, Frederic B.: Cancer of the Mouth, Tongue, and Alimentary Canal, London, 1886.

Johnson, Christopher, T.: Essay on Cancer, London, 1810 (Prize Essay).

Lewers, A. H. N.: Supra-Vaginal Amputation of the Cervix Uteri for Malignant Disease, London, 1888.

Lewis, Daniel: Development of Cancer from Non-malignant Diseases, Reprint from New York Medical Journal, 1883; Cancer and its Treatment, Reprint from American Practitioner, December, 1874; Caustic Treatment of Cancer. New York Medical Record, 1892; A Malignant Tumor in an Umbilical Hernial Sac, New York Medical Record, October 12, 1889.

Marsden, Alexander: New and Successful Mode of Treating Certain Forms of Cancer, London, 1867.

Maunder, C. F.. Tumor of Lower Jaw, London, 1874; Middlesex Hospital Report on Fell's Method, London, 1847.

Mitchell, Robert: Treatise on Cancer Life, London, 1879.

Moore, Chas. H.: Antecedents of Cancer, London, 1865; Cancer of the Tongue, London, 1862.

Norford, Wm.: General Method of Treating Cancerous Tumors, London, 1753.

Nunn, T. W.: Cancer of the Breast, London, 1882.

Paget, Sir James. Lectures on Tumors, London, 1853.

Parker, Willard: Clinical Observations on Cancer—397 Cases of Cancer of the Breast, New York, 1885.

Pearson, John: Practical Observations on Cancerous Complaints, London, 1793.

Pemberton: On Cancer, London, 1867.

Satterthwaite, T. E., and Porter, W. H.: Observations on 100 Cases of Carcinoma, New York, 1879.

Purcell, F. Albert. Cancer and Its Treatment, London, 1881.

Ricketts, B. M.: Ætiology, Diagnosis, and Treatment of Epithelioma, Cincinnati, 1886 (Pamphlet).

Rodman, John: Cancer of Female Breast, Paisley, 1815.

Savory, W. S.: Pathology of Cancer, The Bradshaw Lecture, Royal College of Surgeons, London, 1884.

Snow, Herbert: Clinical Notes on Cancer, London, 1883; Reappearance of Cancer after Operation, London, 1890.

Thin, George. Cancerous Affections of the Skin, London, 1886.

Thompson, E. Symes: Notes on Cases of Tumor in the Mediastinum, London, 1865.

Thompson, Sir Henry: Tumors of the Bladder, London, 1884.

Tuson, E. W.: Structure, Functions, and Diseases of the Female Breast, London, 1846.

Toner Lectores: Smithsonian Institute, Structure of Cancerous Tumors, by J. J. Woodward, 1873.

Velpeau, A.: Diseases of the Breast, Sydenham Society, London, 1856.

Walshe, Walter H.: Nature and Treatment of Cancer, London, 1846.

Warren, John C.: Surgical Operations on Tumors, London, 1839.

Williams, John: Cancer of the Uterus, London, 1888.

The Pepsin Standard Advanced.

There are many varieties of Pepsin in the market, differing widely in purity, activity, and adaptability for therapeutic use.

Whether Pepsin be prescribed with success or failure depends on its quality. The physician prescribing Pepsin should demand in his prescription a pepsin product which he has convinced himself is pure and active, and can be relied upon.

By prolonged investigation of digestive ferments the standard has been again and again advanced. We have succeeded in making a Pepsin capable of digesting 4,000 times its weight of coagulated egg albumen under the conditions of the pharmacopœial test.

This product is prepared by a new and original process which renders it aseptic, free from odor, agreeable in taste to the most sensitive palate, and superior to any pepsin product hitherto made.

In these days when novices and pork-packers are flooding the market with Pepsins, it behooves the careful physician to see that his prescriptions are filled by the product of some reputable manufacturing chemist.

PARKE, DAVIS & CO.,

Manufacturing Chemists,

Detroit, New York, and Kansas City.

IN EXPLANATION

OF

The Physicians' Leisure Library.

We have made a new departure in the publication of medical books. As you no doubt know, many of the large treatises published, which sell for four or five or more dollars, contain much irrelevant matter of no practical value to the physician, and their high price makes it often impossible for the average practitioner to purchase anything like a complete library.

Believing that short practical treatises, prepared by well known authors, containing the gist of what they had to say regarding the treatment of diseases commonly met with, and of which they had made a special study, sold at a small price, would be welcomed by the majority of the profession, we have arranged for the publication of such a series, calling it **The Physicians' Leisure Library.**

This series has met with the approval and appreciation of the medical profession, and we shall continue to issue in it books by eminent authors of this country and Europe, covering the best modern treatment of prevalent diseases.

The series will certainly afford practitioners and students an opportunity never before presented for obtaining a working library of books by the best authors at a price which places them within the reach of all. The books are amply illustrated, and issued in attractive form.

They may be had bound, either in durable paper covers at **25 Cts.** per copy, or in cloth at **50 Cts.** per copy. Complete series of 12 books in sets as announced, at **$2.50,** in paper, or cloth at **$5.00,** postage prepaid. See complete list.

PHYSICIANS' LEISURE LIBRARY

PRICE: PAPER, 25 CTS. PER COPY, $2.50 PER SET; CLOTH, 50 CTS. PER COPY, $5.00 PER SET.

SERIES I.

Inhalers, Inhalations and Inhalants.
By Beverley Robinson, M. D.

The Use of Electricity in the Removal of Superfluous Hair and the Treatment of Various Facial Blemishes.
By Geo. Henry Fox, M. D.

New Medications, Vol. I.
By Dujardin-Beaumetz, M. D.

New Medications, Vol. II.
By Dujardin-Beaumetz, M. D.

The Modern Treatment of Ear Diseases.
By Samuel Sexton, M. D.

The Modern Treatment of Eczema.
By Henry G. Piffard, M. D.

Antiseptic Midwifery.
By Henry J. Garrigues, M. D.

On the Determination of the Necessity for Wearing Glasses.
By D. B. St. John Roosa, M. D.

The Physiological, Pathological and Therapeutic Effects of Compressed Air.
By Andrew H. Smith, M. D.

Granular Lids and Contagious Ophthalmia.
By W. F. Mittendorf, M. D.

Practical Bacteriology.
By Thomas E. Satterthwaite, M. D.

Pregnancy, Parturition, the Puerperal State and their Complications.
By Paul F. Mundé, M. D.

SERIES II.

The Diagnosis and Treatment of Haemorrhoids
By Chas. B. Kelsey, M. D.
Diseases of the Heart, Vol. I.
By Dujardin-Beaumetz, M. D.
Diseases of the Heart, Vol. II.
By Dujardin-Beaumetz, M. D.
The Modern Treatment of Diarrhoea and Dysentery.
By A. B. Palmer, M. D.
Intestinal Diseases of Children, Vol. I.
By A. Jacobi, M. D.
Intestinal Diseases of Children, Vol. II.
By A. Jacobi, M. D.

The Modern Treatment of Headaches.
By Allan McLane Hamilton, M. D.
The Modern Treatment of Pleurisy and Pneumonia.
By G. M. Garland, M. D.
Diseases of the Male Urethra.
By Fessenden N. Otis, M. D.
The Disorders of Menstruation.
By Edward W. Jenks, M. D.
The Infectious Diseases, Vol. I.
By Karl Liebermeister.
The Infectious Diseases, Vol. II.
By Karl Liebermeister.

SERIES III.

Abdominal Surgery.
By Hal C. Wyman, M. D.
Diseases of the Liver
By Dujardin-Beaumetz, M. D.
Hysteria and Epilepsy.
By J. Leonard Corning, M. D.
Diseases of the Kidney.
By Dujardin-Beaumetz, M. D.
The Theory and Practice of the Ophthalmoscope.
By J. Herbert Claiborne, Jr., M. D.
Modern Treatment of Bright's Disease.
By Alfred L. Loomis, M. D.

Clinical Lectures on Certain Diseases of Nervous System.
By Prof. J. M. Charcot, M. D.
The Radical Cure of Hernia.
By Henry O. Marcy, A. M., M. D., L. L. D.
Spinal Irritation.
By William A. Hammond, M. D.
Dyspepsia.
By Frank Woodbury, M. D.
The Treatment of the Morphia Habit.
By Erlenmeyer.
The Etiology, Diagnosis and Therapy of Tuberculosis.
By Prof. H. von Ziemssen.

SERIES IV.

Nervous Syphilis.
By H. C. Wood, M. D.
Education and Culture as correlated to the Health and Diseases of Women.
By A. J. C. Skene, M. D.
Diabetes.
By A. H. Smith, M D.
A Treatise on Fractures.
By Armand Després, M. D.
Some Major and Minor Fallacies concerning Syphilis.
By E. L. Keyes, M .D.
Hypodermic Medication.
By Bourneville and Bricon.

Practical Points in the Management of Diseases of Children.
By I. N. Love, M. D.
Neuralgia.
By E. P. Hurd, M. D.
Rheumatism and Gout.
By F. Le Roy Satterlee, M. D.
Electricity, Its Application in Medicine.
By Wellington Adams, M.D. [Vol.I]
Electricity, Its Application in Medicine.
By Wellington Adams, M.D. [Vol.II]
Auscultation and Percussion.
By Frederick C. Shattuck, M. D.

SERIES V.

Taking Cold.
    By F. H. Bosworth, M. D.

Practical Notes on Urinary Analysis.
    By William B. Canfield, M. D.

Practical Intestinal Surgery. Vol. I.
Practical Intestinal Surgery. Vol. II.
    By F. B. Robinson, M. D.

Lectures on Tumors.
    By John B. Hamilton, M. D., LL. D.

Pulmonary Consumption, a Nervous Disease.
    By Thomas J. Mays, M.D.

Artificial Anaesthetics and Anaesthesia.
    By DeForest Willard, M. D., and Dr. Lewis H. Adler, Jr.

Lessons in the Diagnosis and Treatment of Eye Diseases.
    By Casey A. Wood, M. D.

The Modern Treatment of Hip Disease.
    By Charles F. Stillman, M. D.

Diseases of the Bladder and Prostate.
    By Hal C. Wyman, M. D.

Cancer.
    By Daniel Lewis, M. D.

Insomnia and Hypnotics.
    By Germain Sée.
        Translated by E. P. Hurd, M. D.

SERIES VI.*

The Uses of Water in Modern Medicine. Vol. I.

The Uses of Water in Modern Medicine. Vol. II.
    By Simon Baruch, M. D.

The Electro-Therapeutics of Gynaecology. Vol. I.

The Electro-Therapeutics of Gynaecology. Vol. II.
    By A. H. Goelet, M D.

Cerebral Meningitis.
    By Martin W. Barr, M. D.

Contributions of Physicians to English and American Literature.
    By Robert C. Kenner, M. D.

Gonorrhoea and Its Treatment.
    By G. Frank Lydston, M. D.

Acne and Alopecia.
    By L. Duncan Bulkley, M. D.

Sexual Weakness and Impotence.
    By Edward Martin, M. D.

Fissure of the Anus and Fistula in Ano
    By Dr. Lewis H. Adler, Jr.

Modern Minor Surgical Gynaecology.
    By Edward W. Jenks, M. D.

The Use of the Laryngoscope.
    By J. Solis Cohen, M. D.

---

* To be issued one a month during 1892.

GEORGE S. DAVIS, Publisher,

P. O. Box 470   Detroit, Mich.

BOOKS BY LEADING AUTHORS.

www.ingramcontent.com/pod-product-compliance
Lightning Source LLC
Chambersburg PA
CBHW030603270326
41927CB00007B/1024